Counseling Persons with Communication Disorders and Their Families

COUNSELING PERSONS WITH COMMUNICATION DISORDERS AND THEIR FAMILIES

FOURTH EDITION

David M. Luterman

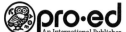
pro·ed
An International Publisher
8700 Shoal Creek Boulevard
Austin, Texas 78757-6897
800/897-3202 Fax 800/397-7633
www.proedinc.com

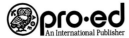

An International Publisher

© 2001, 1996, 1991, 1984 by PRO-ED, Inc.
8700 Shoal Creek Boulevard
Austin, Texas 78757-6897
800/897-3202   Fax 800/397-7633
www.proedinc.com

Library of Congress Cataloging-in-Publication Data

Luterman, David.
    Counseling persons with communication disorders and their families / David M.
    Luterman—4th ed.
       p.   cm.
    Includes bibliographical references and index.
    ISBN 0-89079-876-1
      1. Communicative disorders—Patients—Counseling of. 2. Rehabilitation
    counseling.   I. Title.
    [DNLM: 1. Communication Disorders—therapy. 2. Counseling—methods.
    3. Family
    Therapy. WL 340.2 L973c 2001]
RC428.8 .L87   2001
616.85′8506—dc21
                             2001019614
                             CIP

This book is designed in Goudy.

Printed in the United States of America

2   3   4   5   6   7   8   9   10   05   04   03

*To all clinicians who are
willing to learn from their clients*

Contents

FOREWORD

The last decade has been witness to a revolution in the field of communication disorders. This revolution has been fueled by great advances in medical technology, computer applications, and "high-tech" instrumentation that have become essential tools in the research and treatment of individuals with speech, language, and hearing impairments. In this fourth edition of *Counseling Persons with Communication Disorders and Their Families*, Dr. David M. Luterman makes the case that there also has been another, more quiet, more slowly moving revolution under way, which is certainly not as headline grabbing and flashy as the technology revolution. The terms "raising of consciousness" and "gradual awakening" may more accurately reflect this increasing emphasis in communication disorders and other health-related fields—the awareness that treatment of persons and families with communication disorders should be, at its very core, a psychosocial process. David laments, however, that respect for the human service dimension of communication disorders has been slow in coming and still takes a back seat to a focus on technique and fact-oriented education and training of our students.

David was an early torchbearer of the humanistic and family-centered emphasis in communication disorders, and in this fourth edition he once again persuasively argues that a clinician in communication disorders must be as skilled in working with and supporting people as in applying specific speech–language or audiological assessment or therapy techniques. Furthermore, David clearly communicates that to be an effective clinician, simply having good intentions or being able to empathize with persons and families challenged by a communication disorder is not good enough. A clinician must have a working knowledge of how a disability affects a client and his or her family and of how people generate their own capacities and strategies for coping (both adaptive and maladaptive) under what can be extremely stressful and challenging circumstances.

It is David's respect for the intricacy and complexity of the counseling process that makes his message so special. The prevailing attitude in many health-related professions is that supporting and counseling families is the easy part of the work and should not require special training. After all, we are in this profession because we care about people! Yet, to this day, I continue to be astonished by the "war stories" I hear from families about how the educational or health care system and its professionals (who probably consider themselves well-intentioned and sensitive clinicians) cause as much or greater stress for the family than the disability itself. Furthermore, when clinicians and students discuss the aspect of their work that is most challenging and therefore the source of most professional discomfort and anxiety, working with families and clients on emotional issues such as coping with a disability is invariably at the top of the list. Clearly, we can do much better in working with clients and in training our students.

And this is the message that David infuses throughout this book. David's philosophy of counseling is, at its very core, deeply rooted in an optimistic belief in the human capacity for growth and change. Consistent with his philosophy, this book does not focus on the "affected patient"; the capacity for growth is an issue for systems of human relationships, for professionals, clients, and their families as well as for students in training. For persons and families affected by a disability, David believes that adaptation and coping is largely a process of making meaning out of difficult circumstances and, through this process, finding opportunities for individual and family growth. Because persons and families are so different by virtue of family structure, culture and religion, and specific circumstances surrounding the disability, by necessity, this process is highly subjective and individual. David contends that with the support and guidance of a trained clinician (when needed), the ultimate outcome for a person or family may include empowerment in advocacy and decision making, a greater sense of confidence in coping with challenges, more fulfilling relationships within the family, and in some cases, a reconsideration of one's life path. According to David, a belief in the basic competence of families must underlie the counseling process. For it is with this belief that families can be supported in making (and owning) the most important decisions regarding the affected person and other family members.

This same philosophy is the foundation of David's practices in training professionals in communication disorders and other health-related professions. That is, for effective counseling, the learning of techniques and facts is pointless without the development of a self-generated philosophy consonant with one's own belief system. Thus, David contends that students and professionals need to be able to make mistakes, learn from them, and not be afraid to feel the pain of their clients. The role of mentors and supervisors is to listen, support, and guide but not to provide prescriptions and the "right" answers. It is through this process that students and professionals come to understand and accept their own personal and professional vulnerabilities, and ultimately to better understand those whom they serve. David argues that this process allows clinicians to discard professional masks and scripts in order to truly be able to support the individual and unique human needs of our clients. I have observed that some clinicians may eventually reach this level of "expertise" through years of professional and personal experience. However, as David accurately points out, professional training and constraints inherent in work settings may actually impede such development and encourage a detached working demeanor. Fortunately, through David's writings readers will benefit from the lessons learned from his long and distinguished career as a clinician and professor as well as his own and his family's personal challenges.

For the professional and the student, this book is, in part, about taking risks. The risks include reflecting deeply about how we relate to our clients and their families and whether we take the more difficult path of understanding their pain and grief or remain objectively detached. The risks also include immersing ourselves in a world where simple prescriptions do not work and where there are no cut-and-dried answers. Yet, if we must avoid a "cookbook" approach, we must still be able to move forward and be effective in our relationships with clients and their families. The ultimate risk is to care too much about our life's work and the persons who receive our services. But with these risks comes the greatest reward—the sense that working with clients with communication disorders and their families is an integrated part of our lives and part of our human growth and development, rather than simply a vocation that pays the bills.

For those students and professionals ready to take on these risks in the interest of their own professional and personal growth, I can think of no greater mentor than Dr. David M. Luterman. Largely due to the last 4 years of David's mentorship and friendship, I have grown tremendously in my understanding and therefore in my effectiveness in working with clients and families and with my students. Although I have worked closely with children and families for many years (with the assumption that I was a good clinician), I now experience a challenge and depth in my work that far exceeds what I knew in the past. Those of us who have been able learn directly from David have been very fortunate. It is my sincerest wish that you who read this book also are ready to be nourished by the wisdom and experience that David offers, for I am confident that you will also experience greater fulfillment and challenge in your work.

In the introduction to the second edition of this book, David stated that he would be content if his epitaph read, "He expanded our field by directing our attention to feelings and families." With this fourth edition, I can respond, "He continues to do so, and with great eloquence."

Barry M. Prizant, PhD, CCC-SLP

ACKNOWLEDGMENTS

With the extensive help of my son Dan, I reluctantly entered the 20th century. I think at some point I have offended the technology god because if I can screw up something, I do it. This means I may have to sacrifice my firstborn, but I don't think my daughter will cooperate. Fortunately for both of us, my son has remained patient, and this edition was revised on my newly acquired computer, which I am coming to like when I can get it to behave. My son, however, is currently seeking a support group for the children of technologically challenged parents. He may also need a long vacation after this book is done.

Robin Spencer of PRO-ED was helpful in providing me with materials and support. Like my son, she was immensely patient in guiding me through the intricacies of the computer. She too may need a vacation. Liz Bezera, Emerson College librarian, who is prominently mentioned in my will, gets all sorts of accolades for getting me the necessary materials to make this revision possible.

My wife, Cari, as always, did everything she could to support me. Unfortunately, while this edition was being produced, Cari died. She was a lovely woman who provided me with the support and inspiration I needed to make this book possible.

INTRODUCTION
Fourth Edition (2001)

I have found that one of the gifts of being over 65 is that I have developed the wisdom of using my energy better. Even though I have diminished energy, I seem able to use it more productively than in my youth. One learns the art of pacing; things that seemed hard then are now easy—I just have to nap more. As I get older, I also recognize fully how time limited I am; consequently, I want to use my diminished energy well.

Since the last edition of this text, my wife had a major exacerbation and became quite disabled, necessitating more caregiving on my part. The combination of diminished energy and increased caregiving led to my decision to retire from full-time teaching. I am now an emeritus professor and teach one course, give occasional workshops, and facilitate the parent group at Emerson College. I want to devote more of the time and energy that I have remaining to educating professionals in the field about counseling. There still seems to be a dearth of counseling course being taught in speech and hearing training programs. Crandall (1997), for example, found that only 18% of audiologists took a counseling course in their training program, while Rosenberg (1997) found that 82% of speech pathology graduate students believed they needed more counseling practicum experiences and coursework in their training programs. Rosenberg also believed, as I do, that a counseling course and practicum should be a requirement of CAA-certified programs.

A computer search of the literature has again revealed a dearth of research relating to counseling and communication disorders. Some of the references in this revised edition are 40 years old, reflecting in part on the lack of relevant research and also the timelessness of counseling in its human dimension. As I currently see it in our field, counseling seems to be at a crossroad. I think we have matured enough as a field to recognize the need for addressing the emotional component of communication disorders and its impact on families. On the other hand, we are being driven by managed care and technology to provide a medical model of service delivery that tends to bypass affect counseling. The outcome of this conflict is by no means certain.

Audiology in particular lends itself to a technical base. With the advent of newborn screening, cochlear implants, and sophisticated digital hearing aids, updating on the technical aspects of the profession became essential for audiologists. What good is it, however, to have the technical expertise if we can't communicate effectively with our clients? Counseling needs to be at the forefront of our clinical education and of our research attention; instead, it seems to be an afterthought in most programs. I have long suspected that this is in part due to not having sufficiently trained instructors in our field. This tends to be a self-perpetuting problem, because the current group of clinical instructors did not have any counseling instruction in their training program and therefore are unprepared to teach it.

I am happiest in life when I have windmills at which to tilt. In the words of Eleanor Roosevelt, in life it is easy to grumble about the darkness but much harder to light candles. To that end, I am using monies raised by the college to honor my retirement to fund a series of intensive workshops for college instructors on how to teach counseling. It is my hope that when I have finished in a few years, there will be more counseling teaching infused throughout speech and hearing curricula. I want to add more light to the field.

The writing of the fourth edition of this text was also prompted in part by my desire to provide more information about chronic illness. This is not only a result of my personal experiences and professional practice as I continue to work with well family members of the chronically ill but a recognition on my part that chronic illness presents a huge challenge to our society that is currently not being met. It is increasingly likely that every one of us will be either a caregiver or care recipient in our lifetime. For some this will happen early in their lives, as it did for my wife and me, but for others it will happen late in life. In addition to the chronic illnesses that have always plagued our society, such as lupus, multiple sclerosis, mental illness, and arthritis, we have transformed terminal illnesses into chronic ones. Cancer, AIDS, and heart disease are now chronic illnesses. By *chronic*, I mean those illnesses that are debilitating, have no cure, and will last for the rest of a person's life. My grandfather died at the age of 63. If he were alive today, he would get bypass surgery, live into his 80s, and develop Alzheimer's disease as his son currently has. The chronically ill and their families are threatening to overwhelm our medical facilities, and speech and hearing personnel can expect to be encountering increasing numbers of chronically ill clients and their families. In this revised text, I have substantially increased the amount of material devoted to chronic illness (see chapter 8). In particular, I have written about the relationship between anger and fear and how it reflects on the family systems of the chronically ill.

Of equal concern to me is the change in the counseling paradigm caused by the advent of universal screening of the hearing of newborns. As a result, we have moved from a parent-initiated model of diagnosis to an institution-initiated model. I am not sure the field of audiology has quite grasped the implications of such a change, but they are profound. In the parent-initiated model, the audiologist usually confirms what the parent already knows or suspects and as such can be viewed as an ally. In the institution-initiated model, an unsuspecting parent, 2 days postpartum, is told that his or her child may have a hearing loss. I think that in this model the audiologist will be viewed with hostility and is going to require enhanced counseling skills. I have tried to address this issue in a section of Chapter 5. I think the material in this chapter will be generalizable to all institution-initiated diagnoses and as such should be of interest to speech–language pathologists as well.

In chapter 6, Techniques of Counseling, I have added a section called "counseling caveats" that pulls together material that in previous editions had been scattered throughout the book. I never like to stress the negative, but I have found that counseling is as much a matter of what you do as what you don't do. The essence of counseling as I see it is listening deeply to clients, creating an environment of trust, and then getting out of the way. At one level it is very simple, at another it is quite difficult. It is a matter of students shedding a great many preconceptions that are brought to the counseling relationship. It is my hope that this section will do just that. All other changes in the text are minor.

Personally, in these intervening years I have intensified my involvement with Buddhist philosophy. I find the ideas of *mindfulness* and being in the present and the gentleness of the approach immensely helpful in my personal and professional life. I find the combination of Buddhist and existential thought very helpful in promoting personal growth. I take every opportunity to expose my students to these notions. Hanh's 1998 book, *The Heart of the Buddha's Teaching*, and Kabat-Zinn's 1994 book, *Wherever You Go, There You Are: Mindfulness Meditation in Everyday Life*, very helpful in shaping my thoughts. Prior to meditating with my counseling class, I read portions of the latter book. The manual for the classroom teacher that accompanies this text, which is available from the publisher, presents some ideas for integrating both Buddhist and existential ideas into the classroom.

I also have found the work of Cassell attractive. His 1991 book, *The Nature of Suffering*, presents some interesting thoughts concerning the transcendance that often accompanies pain and suffering. This is something I have noticed in both my personal and professional lives. People often ask me how I have been able to stay professionally active so long admidst so much pain and suffering. The answer is that I tell parents I will share their pain if they will share with me their joy and growth in dealing with their child's problem. These are the moments of grace that make this profession worthwhile.

In life one seldom knows when a "last" has come. I know that while preparing several previous revisions of this text I felt that it was the last time, only to pick up pen again (this time it has been laboriously hunting and pecking my way through on my new computer). At this time, it feels like a last. I have left intact the introductions to the previous editions of this text. The interested reader can use them to understand the evolution of my thinking; the uninterested reader can go right to the text. Both readers may want to wait for the movie.

Third Edition (1996)

It is time to pick up my pen again—perhaps for the last time—prompted in large part by the recent article in *Asha* by Culpepper, Mendel, and McCarthy (1994), which indicated that there has been little change in the number of counseling courses within our training programs since their last survey 8 years ago. A computer search of our literature also indicates almost nothing new on counseling issues, yet almost everyone in training programs, according to Culpepper et al., believes that counseling is an important component of effective therapy and should be basic to the training of clinicians. It seems that for us as a profession counseling is much like Mark Twain's quip about the weather: Everybody talks about it, but nobody does anything about it. I have long suspected that the reason for the dearth of literature and coursework is the lack of experienced teachers within our profession who have the dual knowledge of counseling process and communication disorders. The majority of our programs that offer a counseling course still offer it as a nondepartmental elective (Culpepper, et al.). This indicates to me that we don't have the teachers within our profession who have the requisite skills and knowledge.

One of my major justifications for writing this new edition is to make the text more teacher friendly in the hope that more instructors will be emboldened to adopt this text and offer a counseling course. In keeping with this rationale, I have also written a manual for teaching a course in counseling; this manual is available from the publisher. And, if teachers don't offer a specific course, I hope they will infuse their communication disorders curriculum with counseling notions. Since the last edition of this text, I have been in contact with several instructors at other universities who are trying to teach counseling. Many of them have been teaching from a technique orientation, using role-playing class activities and detailing therapists' responses to specific client situations. I think trying to teach counseling from a technique orientation is counterproductive. It is easy to teach this way, and students are happy because it gives them a structure on which to hold; however, approaching counseling from a technique orientation reduces the naturalness of the interpersonal encounter, which is, I believe, the heart of good counseling. Students with a technique orientation are left self-conscious and mechanical in their responses to client feelings. Good counseling needs to be seamless, and the process must be natural to the personality of the clinician. I am reminded of the story of the annual golf tournament that was held in a small town. Each year one man would beat out another until the second-place finisher gave the winner a book entitled *How to Play Golf*. After that, he won every year.

I have been teaching a counseling course at Emerson College for the past 15 years, and I have also taught intensive counseling courses at several universities. I am convinced that the most fruitful way to teach counseling is through a personal growth paradigm. The course itself needs to be a genuine encounter between the instructor and students to encourage personal growth of the students. In short, the instructor is always modeling good counseling interactions by using the students' life experiences as the raw material for learning. To be sure, there is a body of cognitive material that needs to be learned. At the least, our students need to be exposed to it, and I have left intact in this edition all cognitive material from previous editions, adding to it where appropriate.

The content and the specifics of counseling technique, however, should not be the major focus of the course. Effective counseling (and good therapy) is basically a right-brain experience. We need to be able to operate from our intuitive center. Too often our teaching is of the left-brain variety, whereby we teach students academic performance without clinical competency. Very often it isn't until students let go of what they have learned in school that they become truly effective clinicians. Our goal as educators must be to give students a solid knowledge base that is integrated with and guided by their clinical intuitions and feelings. We must give our students permission to be authentic human beings in a genuine encounter with their clients. The dilemma for the teacher is how to balance right- and left-brain teaching. I hope this edition of the text will provide help for the instructor in doing just that.

I have also finally completed writing the book describing my family's struggle with multiple sclerosis (*In the Shadows: Living and Coping with a Loved One's Chronic Illness*, 1995). This book was a long time in the writing (nearly 10 years), as I kept putting it aside to work on other projects. The writing for me was also very painful; the story was everchanging as we moved and are moving further down the disability path. In writing that book I delved deeply into the disability literature and how chronic illness of a significant adult affects families. This hard-won information is now incorporated into a very much-revised Chapter 8. In the previous edition, that chapter was very much skewed to families with young children with disabilities; it is now in better balance.

What I have come to realize in an increasing way is how important marriage—whether it be spousal or parental—is to the eventual success of our clients. Working with families of newly diagnosed deaf children has shown me that the children who turn out best are the products of a strong marriage; I have also found that the adults with disabilities who are coping most successfully are the ones with strong marriages. In the third edition, especially in the revised chapter on families, I have addressed marriage as a key component of successful coping for our clients.

Once again, several gurus have influenced me strongly through their books: Gardner's 1991 book, *The Unschooled Mind,* in which he makes a strong case for experiential learning, has influenced my thinking about how best to teach counseling. Nuland's 1994 book, *How We Die,* and Levine's 1982 book, *Who Dies,* have reinforced for me again the idea of how time limited we all are, and therefore how fragile and precious life is. These notions are vital to the success of the counselor. Levine's other book, *A Gradual Awakening* (1979), has helped me learn to meditate and find the centering calm that enables me to listen, which I believe is the essence of good counseling. I have recently begun to bring meditation into the classroom, with generally favorable reactions from the students.

My preoccupation with death is not morbid, but living with death awareness for me means that I do not postpone living; my wife's illness has also taught me that. Recently, I passed my 60th birthday, and the inexorable progression of my wife's illness and her increasing disability have restricted the time and energy I can devote to professional endeavors. I can sense the closing down of my very active involvement in professional affairs. I hope to continue teaching and doing occasional workshops, and it is my fondest wish that this text should become the stimulus for the creation of more counseling courses in our field that are taught by instructors with a background in communication disorders.

Second Edition (1991)

An author never really knows when a book is finished: A bell doesn't go off, and nobody taps you on the shoulder. More often than not, you are just exhausted and fed up with the material. (Apollinaire said, "Novels are never finished; they are only abandoned.") Such was the case with the first edition of this book. I had just felt written out, although I knew as I was writing the chapter on the family that here was a rich lode of material that needed to be mined at a later date. The material on the family led me into literature seldom used in our field and subsequently became the book *Deafness in the Family* (1987).

During the intervening years since the publication of the first edition, my wife Cari developed multiple sclerosis. We actually knew she had it at the time I was writing the first edition of this book, but it was relatively benign and was not really interfering with our very busy lives. Five years after the publication of the first edition, the disease had progressed to the point where it was and has become a very important and dominating factor in our lives. This prompted me to look at how people, especially well family members, can cope with chronic, progressive illness of a loved one; it was a study of powerlessness in the face of diseases such as multiple sclerosis, Alzheimer's, arthritis, lupus, and diabetes. This study became the as-yet unpublished manuscript *The Shadow People*. This study brought me outside the field of communication disorders and made me realize again how universal the counseling and coping issues are. My experiences in writing these two more recent books after completing the first edition of this text gave me much more material that needed to be incorporated into this second edition.

In addition, several studies have been published since the first edition, notably the studies of Martin, George, O'Neal, and Daly (1987) and Williams and Derbyshire (1982), which indicated that audiologists in particular were ineffective in their counseling (although I suspect that if the same studies were done with speech pathologists, similar results would occur). The need for counseling skills in our profession is almost self-evident, yet somehow we are still failing to effectively train students in these counseling skills. McCarthy, Culpepper, and Lucks (1986), in their survey of departmental chairs, found that only 12% of the respondents felt that training programs were effective in training students in counseling. As a consequence of our ineptitude, many functioning clinicians are bereft of good counseling abilities and are therefore not very effective in what they do.

Counseling cuts across all disorders—it is both universal and timeless, based as it is on good interpersonal relationships. Once we get away from disorder-specific and content-based thinking, we can see the commonality of our universe. Under the disability skin we are all brothers and sisters, and it makes no difference whether we counsel people who stutter, parents of children who are deaf, people with aphasia, or well family members of people who are chronically ill. We are dealing with loss, and the grief response seems universal in our culture. Grieving people need to be in a relationship with a responsive and caring professional who is equipped with good counseling skills.

As stated in the introduction to the first edition, which bears repeating here, it is not the purpose of this book to make "counselors" of speech pathologists and audiologists—to supplant the work of social workers or psychologists in a clinical setting. Rather it is to help the professionals who work with individuals with communication disorders to incorporate some of the knowledge and skills of trained counselors in order to enhance their own clinical effectiveness. In short, the purpose is to make us clinicians as opposed to technicians, to move us beyond the narrow technical base of our field into a much more expansive one that allows and encourages speech pathologists and audiologists to work with and be comfortable about the myriad of feelings that accompany a communication disorder. We are working with people who are emotionally upset, not necessarily emotionally disordered, and, as such, we need to develop the skills to deal with emotional adjustment issues and family issues.

I also would like to draw attention to the well family members. When there is a communication disorder in a family, everyone is affected by it, and it therefore becomes the responsibility of the speech pathologist and the audiologist to work with the needs of all members of the family.

A communication disorder always exists within a "family" context. It cannot be confined to a single individual because the disorder manifests itself only within the milieu of a relationship. For us to be effective, to be clinicians, we must examine and deal with the whole relationship. I have found in my professional life that by working intimately with parents of deaf children, if you take good care of the parents, the children will do well. This admonition applies equally well to the chronically ill; if you take good care of the spouse and other family members, the identified patient also will do well. Failure to deal with family needs almost invariably limits therapeutic effectiveness. In this text "client" refers as much to the family member as it does to the identified person with a communication disorder.

When my professional epitaph gets written, and I hope it is not yet for a while, I would like it to say, "He expanded our field by directing our attention to feelings and families." In this new edition, which I hope will appeal to both the student in training and the practicing clinician, the reader will find the following changes:

Chapter 1 is an entirely new chapter reflecting the literature of our ineffectiveness as counselors and presenting my own definition and model of counseling.

Chapter 2 on contemporary theories of counseling is a compilation of material that is in the first edition. My love affair with existentialism and its application to our field continues unabated. I still value humanism very highly, and I have a grudging respect for the potent contributions that behaviorism and the rational/emotive approaches can make in our field.

Chapter 3 is the only chapter unchanged from the first edition. I think Erikson's life cycle model is such a powerful and universal tool that students and clinicians need to be exposed to it. It is also very useful for understanding relationship building.

Chapter 4 on the emotions is material that was scattered throughout the first edition. In this chapter the material has been rewritten and recast to reflect how emotions can lead to self-defeating behavior and, if not handled well by the clinicians, can undermine any effective therapy. In particular, it is the nonunderstanding of the denial mechanism and its role in the coping process by us as a profession that limits our effectiveness.

Chapter 4 also contains new material on coping that reflects my research with the families of the chronically ill. Here the clinician will find a model of the coping process and techniques for coping that can be applied to a broad clinical caseload.

Chapter 5 on the diagnostic process is a new one and reflects my increasing awareness of the importance of the imprinting that occurs in the initial contact between clients and professionals. The diagnostic process can be and should be handled in such a way as to minimize the denial mechanism and to facilitate all subsequent client–professional interactions.

Chapter 6 on the techniques of counseling is an expanded chapter that gives more material for the clinician to practice effective listening as well as suggestions for refraining, which I am increasingly seeing as a very useful clinical intervention when used judiciously. I am also including "hypothetical" families in this chapter. This was a technique that I used and wrote about in my very first book. I think this can be a useful case-study approach for beginning clinicians as well as a technique to stimulate and direct group discussion.

Chapter 7 on the group process is slightly expanded from the first edition. I stand very committed to the group process as a strong educational vehicle. I want very much to encourage and support the development of more groups within our field. To this end, we need to develop competence and confidence in group facilitating. I ardently hope this chapter does both.

Chapter 8 on the family is completely rewritten and markedly expanded, reflecting material that was in *Deafness in the Family*. In particular, I think the material on the optimal and successful families will be of use to the practicing clinician.

Chapter 9 is my attempt to look ahead for our field and to see how counseling skills will enrich our growth as a profession and in training students.

It is now time for me to "abandon" this manuscript. I think I have shared all I know at this point, and although nobody is tapping me on the shoulder and no bells are going off, I know it is time for me to stop. At this point I feel good that this volume accurately reflects my 30 years of clinical and teaching experience.

First Edition (1984)

More than 20 years ago I started my career as a clinical audiologist. At that time I thought I was interested in the precision and surety that working with machines seemed to give. I soon realized that I was not a "machine person" but rather a "people person" and that the audiologic machinery was getting in the way of my relating to people. It was with some trepidation that I decided to come out from behind my audiometer and relate as a person rather than as a professional. The first outward manifestation of my slowly evolving inner changes was the willingness to wear nonwhite shirts; soon I went tieless. A few years later, I abandoned suits and sports jackets—the uniform of the male professional. Most recently I have given up all titles and prefer people to call me by my first name. These changes took more than 10 years to accomplish.

Rather than make a radical change in my life, I sought another way of relating to the hearing-impaired population. It became apparent to me that parents of children who were severely hearing impaired were not being treated well. I was the clinical audiologist who confirmed the parents' suspicion that they had a child who was, who proceeded to talk extensively about a course of action, and who then referred them to an educational facility. My information giving was designed to keep me in control of the situation, to conform to the parents' expectations and my own perception of what a professional was, and to distance the parents from their feelings, which I did not know how to handle. It also became apparent to me, on subsequent visits, that the needs of parents were not being met by either the educational facilities or by me. So with a great deal of naïveté, I decided in 1965 to begin a parent-centered nursery program at Emerson College in Boston. In addition to a nursery and language therapy for the children, the Emerson program provided a once-a-week session designed as a parent support group, which I led. I decided early to forego my information-providing function (I had to—I had only a small number of set speeches and I was committing myself to 30 sessions with the parents) and spent much of each session listening to the parents. The program has continued to the present day and has afforded me a great opportunity to grow both personally and professionally. Out of my experience came a book describing the program in detail with procedures for counseling parents of children with hearing impairments (Luterman, 1979).

I found that as I allowed more affect (feelings) to enter into these relationships (I could, for example, allow the parents to cry), listened more, and dealt less with content, people learned more. When the information was spaced over time, and when I allowed parents to work through their very normal feelings about having a child who was deaf, the parents could absorb and retain the information I was providing. I realized in my audiologist mode that all those brilliant set speeches that I had been delivering had not been retained by the parents anyway, as on subsequent visits I found that parents were asking me questions that I thought I had already covered adequately. I also discovered that people were not as fragile as I had thought (actually, it was my own fragility I had been worrying about) and that they could defend themselves quite well against my insensitivities and all-too-frequent lack of skill. As long as I remained a caring, listening person, growth occurred within the relationship. I seemed to serve parents much better when I did not function in the traditional information-providing mode. As an added bonus, I found that my professional boredom was replaced by excitement.

During the past several years, I have been teaching courses and giving workshops on counseling issues to working audiologists and speech pathologists. These experiences have made me aware that attitudes have not changed very much regarding counseling in the 20-odd years since I started working as a professional. Counseling as practiced by most audiologists and speech–language pathologists still seems to be of the information-imparting or advice-giving variety (i.e., the medical or quasimedical model). If the relationship between the professional and the individual with communication disorders gets into the emotional area, the audiologist/speech–language pathologist becomes uncomfortable and tends to hide behind content or to refer the patient to a social worker or psychologist. The information-providing role, however, is not satisfactory over the long run. One is apt to be bored delivering all the set speeches accumulated over a working lifetime. Professionals dealing with communication disorders who wish to change tend, after a few years of information providing, to seek other ways of relating to those they are helping; hence the attendance at workshops on counseling.

Those professionals who do not find another way of relating tend to "burn out" quickly. The burnout rate in our field is quite high; 43% of surveyed speech–language pathologists reported moderate to severe burnout, which involved a loss of concern for the feelings of their clients (Miller & Potter, 1982).

I think it is generally acknowledged that counseling skills are an important concomitant of the well-trained speech pathologist, yet little formal training is provided in educational programs. An examination of graduate catalogs indicates few courses offered specifically on counseling for the speech clinician, nor is a course in counseling required for certification by the American Speech-Language-Hearing Association.

Counseling skills, when they are obtained by graduate clinicians, seem to be obtained informally through students' observation of other clinicians or almost incidentally picked up as students acquire specific skills in altering speech and language behavior. Too many of our students are leaving training programs with a very limited view of their capacity to involve themselves in intensive relationships with their clients.

This book was initiated—as I suspect many texts are—when I agreed to teach a course on counseling individuals with communication disorders and found that there was no single, satisfactory text. The ultimate purpose of this book is to demystify the counseling experience for the professional working within the field of communication disorders. It is my hope that as a result of reading this book, clinicians will feel more comfortable in allowing the affect that is a normal concomitant of having a communication disorder to emerge in their clinical interactions. I hope this book will provide some insight into relationship building and how it affects the counseling process. By allowing more affect to occur in the relationships, speech–language pathologists and audiologists will find that their information-providing role will be enhanced and they will therefore be much more effective. I think they will also obtain more job satisfaction.

This text is not intended to supplant the clinical use of social workers or psychologists: They are trained professionals whose skills will be needed within a comprehensive speech–language and hearing program. I hope, however, that this text will lead to a modified use of professional counselors so that they can provide support and ongoing inservice training to speech–language pathologists/audiologists as they deal with the normal emotions surrounding a communication disorder and provide direct service to clients with emotional disorders who may also have a communication disorder.

During the past several years I have come to value highly the use of Erik Erikson's stages of growth as a means of understanding both the difficulties of the individual with communication disorder and the development of a counseling relationship. Recently I have come across the writings of Irvin Yalom on existential issues in psychotherapy, which I believe have far-reaching implications for the field of communication disorders. This text reflects my expanded appreciation of both Erikson and Yalom.

I have devoted a chapter to group counseling, as I feel that this area of counseling can be better utilized by the speech and hearing clinician. I have also devoted more space to the denial mechanism than I did in my previous book because I have come to see more clearly how the difficulties of the professional in handling the complex issue of denial limit effective counseling.

In writing this book I have drawn heavily on my own experience in the field of deafness and in particular on my work with parents. I have made no attempt to delineate content counseling for specific speech disorders as I assume that the well-trained speech–language pathologist has this information. Counseling skills are applicable to all disorders once the professional acquires them. By extension, much of the material is also appropriate for other disabling conditions that do not necessarily involve a communication disorder. I hope that this book is of use to any professional working with the communication disorders who wishes to get beyond the information-providing role.

CHAPTER

COUNSELING BY THE SPEECH–LANGUAGE PATHOLOGIST AND AUDIOLOGIST

As an aspiring audiologist in training, I learned that counseling was something one did after obtaining a careful case history and administering diagnostic tests. Counseling was always information based and involved an explanation of the audiogram and recommendations for follow-through. I don't recall if as graduate students we were given an explicit injunction not to deal with the client's feelings, but we behaved as though we were. If a client displayed feelings (e.g., by crying), we were to refer the client to the clinical psychologist. The message I received in my training program was that client affect was the province of social workers and psychologists and that counseling by audiologists and speech–language pathologists was to be information based. This was essentially a medical model of counseling and reflected, I think, a desire to keep the field of communication disorders as a distinct entity as well as to avoid infringing on other professions. It also reflected the lack of counseling training in graduate programs at that time. In addition, staying with content was professionally safe: With content, students could control the interactions; emotions were unpredictable and therefore potentially disruptive. With the medical model, students could adopt an attitude of detached concern and proceed to control the clinical interaction by delivering set speeches.

The medical model, at least among audiologists, remains the prevalent counseling approach. In a questionnaire study of 226 audiologists, Flahive and White (1982) found that a great proportion of the audiologists' time was spent in informational counseling as opposed to personal adjustment counseling. The audiologists also reported that in their training programs they had been exposed to much more informational counseling (90%) than personal adjustment counseling (10%).

Many audiologists and speech–language pathologists receive no training in counseling. McCarthy et al. (1986) surveyed training programs accredited by the American Speech-Language-Hearing Association (ASHA). They found that only 40% of the programs offered a course in counseling within the department (36% had an out-of-department course and 23% had no offering at all). The most telling finding was that although the overwhelming majority of respondents felt that counseling was an important skill for speech pathologists to acquire, only 12% of the respondents felt that training programs were effective in training students in counseling. As noted in the introduction to this book, a repeat of this survey (Culpepper et al., 1994) indicated little change in the number of counseling courses offered in our training programs.

This lack of training is reflected in an increasing body of information indicating that audiologists are not effective in their counseling. Williams and Derbyshire (1982) questioned 25 parents of children with severe and profound hearing impairment under the age of 11 years within 1 year of their having been seen by an audiologist. The results of the questionnaire study and personal interviews were startling and rather disheartening. The responses indicated that 84% of the parents were unable to understand all of the information they had been given, 72% did not know what a hearing loss would mean to their children, and 64% did not have a realistic appreciation of how the hearing loss would affect their own lives. When asked by the investigators to restate the audiologist's explanations of the implications of hearing loss, 40% could not do so at all and 24% attempted explanations that the investigators felt were incorrect. Martin, Krueger, and Bernstein (1990) conducted a questionnaire survey of 35 adults with hearing impairment shortly after they had had an audiological examination and had received content counseling from the audiologist. The authors concluded that "even when audiologists feel they have adequately covered all of the information during the audiological examination, the hearing-impaired adults' knowledge of this information is still lacking" (p. 32). Incredibly, not one respondent in their survey knew what an audiogram was after having just completed the examination.

In a national survey of audiologists and parents of children with hearing impairment, Martin et al. (1987) found that there were many important dissimilarities in the perceptions of audiologists and parents, primary among which were the differences in the acceptance of deafness and in who should provide the counseling. In an unpublished master's thesis, Lerner (1988) interviewed in depth the parents of a young child who was deaf (diagnosed at age 2 months) and the audiologists who had tested the child and counseled the parents. The parents were well-educated professionals—the father was a physician and the mother was a computer programmer. Both audiologists had doctoral degrees and 10 to 12 years of experience. The audiologists believed that they had done a good job of conveying the necessary information. The parents, on the other hand, were very dissatisfied, feeling that jargon was inappropriately used. For example, they felt the term "severe to profound" in describing their child's hearing loss was useless to them. (How often do audiologists use that terminology so casually?) What the parents most remembered was the tone of the comments, which to them was negative and pessimistic.

In my own clinical experience, this reaction is fairly typical of parents of children who are newly diagnosed as being deaf. When they leave the audiologist's office, they feel very confused and emotionally hurt and have not absorbed much of the informational counseling that was provided. Parents invariably remember irrelevant details—the dress the audiologist was wearing or the color of a tie—and although they retain little content, they always remember the emotional tone set by the audiologist—whether he or she was upbeat, hopeful, and emotionally supportive or cold and factual.

Perhaps the crowning blow to our counseling egos was delivered by the study conducted by Haas and Crowley (1982). The results of their survey indicated that parents of children who are deaf felt that the professional who provided them with the most meaningful information was the educator rather than the audiologist.

Certainly, some effective counseling is being provided within our field, and at times providing information is very appropriate. The audiologists in the Lerner (1988) study did have many successes; at the same time, however, we can be more effective as a profession if we are sensitive to the emotional state of our clients and feel comfortable in allowing affect to be a component of our clinical interactions.

It would seem that I am picking on the counseling skills of audiologists because all of the previous studies detailing failure of counseling were related to hearing disorders. Unfortunately, there are no comparable studies in speech pathology. These studies badly need to be done. I suspect they will yield comparable results if the information provided by speech–language pathologists is offered without recourse or sensitivity to the emotional state of the client.

In addition to counseling by informing, many professionals in our field counsel by persuading, which is a very seductive model of counseling. The underlying assumption of this approach is that "I as a professional have all of this information and experience. You as the client are ignorant of so many things that you need to know; therefore, I can make a better decision for you than you can for yourself." This approach often confirms clients' perceptions of their own limitations; they generally are feeling so inadequate and overwhelmed by the problem at hand that they often acquiesce to our arguments and recommendations and let the "doctor" decide. This is particularly true in the counseling of hearing parents of children who are deaf. A blatant example of counseling by persuasion can be found in an article by Dee (1981) in which she described her total communication program for parents of children with hearing impairment. (It could just as well have been an oral program. The issue here is the counseling style, not the methodology.)

> Most hearing parents of deaf infants need considerable help and guidance in developing clear and honest convictions about the real values of the total communication approach in the life of a deaf infant and his/her family. Even after their first pleasurable experience with total communication, during family sessions, when they have learned to use the simultaneous method to achieve a warm and loving communicative interaction with their infant, some of our parents will continue to undergo periods of doubt, uncertainty and even occasional resistance. Parents might also be struggling against non-supportive and/or antagonistic attitudes toward manual communication expressed by grandparents, relatives and friends. Furthermore, almost all parents cannot help but be vulnerable to the highly persuasive claims of the oralist. It is essential, therefore, to provide parents in total communication programs with a strong and convincing rationale for continuing to use this communication mode. A parent education program can provide yearlong opportunities for exploring and evaluating all that is 'total' about total communication and for expanding and strengthening parental understanding of and belief in the emotional and educational gains that are the rewards of a total communication way of life. (Dee, 1981, p. 15)

This mode of counseling assumes that parents are weak and incapable of effective decision making: People generally conform to our expectations of them.

I, too, can recall persuading clients. A druggist with a very significant hearing loss once came in with his wife because she had been nagging him to get a hearing aid. Both the wife and I ganged up on him to persuade him to get an aid; she was arguing about how hard it was to live with him and I was arguing about how difficult it must be at work and how hazardous it might be for his customers. He finally agreed to get the aid, but a follow-up call 6 months later indicated that the hearing aid was in the drawer most of the time and the wife was as frustrated and angry as ever.

❀ Counseling by persuasion is usually a poor approach because the clients never "own" their behavior. It also diminishes the client with the implicit assumption that the client isn't smart enough to figure out things for him- or herself. Clients do not take responsibility for having made the decision; the responsibility remains with the professional. My own experience in dealing with deafness has been that parents who have been persuaded to learn sign language with their children are the ones who drop out of sign class early and seldom use total communication at home; likewise, clients who are persuaded to get a hearing aid seldom wear it on a regular basis. True change comes from the inside when the client has made a decision and is willing to commit to it.

The second problem with counseling by persuasion is that it reinforces the client's feelings of inadequacy. It becomes a confirmation of the client's own felt inability to make a good decision and therefore the decision is to "trust the professional." This creates the dependent client—the one who is less apt to take any initiatives or responsibilities for solving the problem. The work is all left to the speech pathologist or audiologist who "knows better." This situation also tends to create fanatical parents—those who have been "brainwashed" and must now believe ardently in a particular approach, which has to be right because they have no other recourse, not having developed any confidence in themselves or in their decision-making skills. These are parents who do not think reflectively—they just believe. This is neither good education nor good counseling.

These two counseling approaches—counseling by informing and counseling by persuading—are not mutually exclusive. There are components of both in most inadequate counseling sessions. After first informing the client of test results, we often set about convincing him or her of what to do about the data. A combination of informing and persuading counseling strategies can be very potent. When we overwhelm with information, we also undermine the client's confidence, leaving him or her very vulnerable to being persuaded.

A third approach to counseling clients is the one I prefer: counseling by listening and valuing. In this approach, the clients are seen as possessing the wisdom to ultimately make good decisions for themselves, and the professionals are seen as people who have the specialized knowledge to help illuminate the possibilities for them. Counseling must always increase possibilities. By listening and valuing the client, the professional bolsters the client's confidence so that good decisions ultimately are made. For me, counseling is a mutually educative process that allows for the exchange of both information and affect. The aim of counseling is to help the client become better able to contend successfully with the specific problem at hand. Counseling as practiced by speech–language pathologists and audiologists should be problem centered for individuals who are emotionally upset by the issue at hand. This is opposed to psychotherapy, the province of specially trained professionals who are dealing with people who have chronic life adjustment problems. Many of the skills needed by both counselors and psychotherapists overlap considerably. It is the nature of the client and the nature of the problem that differ.

To be successful in counseling, we speech and hearing professionals must help clients to become more *congruent*. A person's ability to function effectively in the world is a combination of the intellectual abilities (cognition) by which we process data and the emotions (affect) by which we intuit the world. When one is congruent, one has equal access to intellect and to affect and decision making becomes easier because of an increased awareness of who and what one is. When a person is able to respond to a situation with both intellect and emotion, the behavior is always self-enhancing. Total congruence is an idealized state for most of us and is achieved only at very special peak moments in life, but we as professionals need to be always striving to become more congruent in our lives, as we need to always be working to increase client congruence.

Most people tend to have their own particular style of internal organization. Some people are high in intellect and short on affect; others are inclined to approach the world and personal problems from a feeling orientation, with little recourse to information. Invariably these opposites are attracted to each other as they seek to achieve congruence via relationship, if not in the world. This is important for us to note when we are counseling couples; invariably they will be approaching the situation from different perspectives. The stress of a crisis, which often occurs around a communication disorder, tends to push people further into their particular orientation. Individuals who are cognitively oriented want "just the facts," and individuals who are affect oriented are so full of emotion that they cannot deal with any facts; obviously this presents unique problems for the counselor.

To be effective at counseling, we must allow the person who is affect oriented to vent feelings so that he or she can begin to process the information that is needed, and we must help the person who is intellectually oriented gain access to feelings to become more congruent. This listening, and valuing approach to counseling mandates that the speech and hearing professional be comfortable with the client's feelings and develop skills to elicit them. I have found that this counseling approach is very often frightening to many professionals in our field. If we are not informing and we are not persuading, who are we? Gregory (1983) described the problem well when he commented about counseling persons who stutter:

> It may be that giving information expresses dominance and giving direction is related to manipulation and control. Whereas we may view listening and attempting to understand as being indecisive and uncertain. For whatever reason many student clinicians and professional speech–language pathologists seem to find it easier to be a provider of information and direction. (p. 10)

The idea of allowing feelings to be expressed and eliciting them is also frightening because of our mistaken belief that clients are emotionally fragile and somehow we can hurt them by allowing them to talk about and display their feelings. If one thinks about it, how can we hurt people by listening to them and valuing them? E. Webster (1977) said it well when she wrote the following:

> If counseling means the imposition of prescriptions without care for the person for whom they are prescribed, one may indeed do damage. The non-accepting, non-compassionate clinician runs the risk of hurting parents, so does the one who focuses concern on the child to the exclusion of concern for the parents. The speech pathologist or audiologist who leaves to others the interpretation of the information his field has to offer may do parents great harm. The same can be said for the clinician with limited knowledge who gives faulty information.
>
> On the other hand, it is virtually impossible for one person to damage another by listening to him, by trying to understand what the world looks like to him, by permitting him to express what is in him, and by honestly giving him the information he needs. In this view of counseling, the clinician serves as an accepting listener. He delays his judgement and tries to accept parents as they are and as they will become. (p. 337)

It is my hope that this text will help the speech and hearing professional expand his or her viewpoint to include other ways of relating to clients beyond informing and persuading. With that in mind, we need first to examine current theory and how that theory has implications for our field; then we can look at the applications of a listening and valuing orientation to counseling clients.

CHAPTER

CONTEMPORARY THEORIES OF COUNSELING

There is an Indian parable about some blind men and an elephant. Each man held on to a piece of the elephant and when asked to describe the beast, gave a very different version of the animal. The blind man who clutched the tail described the elephant as small, thin, and snakelike. The man clutching the leg described the elephant as very large and solid, whereas the one who had the trunk thought an elephant was flexible and strong. The point of the parable is that a person's view of reality depends on which part he or she is grasping and that perhaps each of us has a limited view of reality at any given time.

A clinician trying to help a client manage change is much like one of the blind men in the parable. Clinicians operate from a theoretical framework that gives them a particular view of the "elephant." In practice, I think successful clinicians are eclectic in that they can and do mix their views and are always evaluating which particular view is most useful in facilitating a therapeutic goal that fits the client context. Most counselors, however, still operate from a central tendency—that is, their theory of the therapeutic process—which provides the organizing principles by which they tend to see client behavior. With that in mind, I want to examine the possible applications of four contemporary theories of counseling to the field of communication disorders: behavioral, humanistic, existentialist, and cognitive.

Behavioral Counseling

The behavioral model of counseling originated in the work of John Watson, with roots going back to Ivan Pavlov and his work with dogs and conditioned responses. Behaviorists concentrate on the strictly observable, with an emphasis on external, environmental influences. (This emphasis was in sharp contrast to the subjectivity of the Freudian movement, which was beginning to invade U.S. psychology around 1950, after many Freudians immigrated to the United States to avoid the Holocaust during World War II.) The leading proponent of behaviorism in the United States was B. F. Skinner. His seminal work *Science and Human Behavior* (1953) became the basis of the clinical application of behaviorist notions to the alteration of maladaptive human behavior. Prior to that time, behaviorism had pretty much been confined to academic laboratory exploration using experimental animals (mainly mice and pigeons; Rimm & Cunningham, 1985).

Skinner contended that human behavior is shaped by the environment that "operates" on it: If a particular behavior is rewarded—that is, reinforced by the environment—that behavior will be repeated. Reinforcement is either positive, as when a reward is given when the desired behavior is elicited, or negative, as when an aversive stimulus is removed as a consequence of the individual's behavior. (Negative reinforcement is not to be confused with punishment, in which an aversive stimulus such as an electric shock is applied as a consequence of behavior.) The reinforcement, whether positive or negative, must be applied according to a precise schedule. The timing must be exact so that the person associates the reinforcement with the behavior (this does not have to be conscious, as we shall see shortly), and the reinforcer must be either desirable to the individual or aversive enough to cause the behavior to change. Strict behavioral psychologists believe that there is no freedom or choice: All behavior is a product of external reinforcements.

The behavioral therapist designs therapy based on the observable. This is basically an "engineering" model of facilitating change in that a goal is set and the task is broken down into a series of small steps. Each successive approximation is achieved by the judicious application of reinforcement. As long as the reinforcer is appropriate, the timing of its application is precise, and the desired behavior is within the physiological capabilities of the organism (e.g., one cannot get an elephant to fly, Dumbo notwithstanding), then the behavior will change.

There is a story, perhaps apocryphal, that is told about a psychology professor who was lecturing his class on operant conditioning techniques. On its own, the class decided to condition the professor. Every time he moved to the right, the class would sit up, take notes, and appear to be interested (powerful rein-forcers to any professor). As soon as he moved to the left, they would slump in their seats and appear to be quite inattentive. It was not long before he was lec-turing from the doorway situated at the far right of the room. When the class got bored with this, they modified his behavior by reinforcing any movement to the left, and pretty soon he was lecturing from the window. The professor, sophisticated as he was, responded much like any pigeon or mouse in a Skinner box, the apparent victim of the reinforcement schedule maintained by the class.

The fact that the behavior of humans can be changed as a result of the sys-tematic application of reinforcement can be demonstrated both in laboratory conditions and in actual living conditions. This approach has diverse applica-tions to speech pathology and audiology.

Applications to Communication Disorders

Behaviorism is a very attractive way of dealing with the deviant behaviors one encounters in a speech and hearing clinic. It provides a structured framework by which the therapist (especially the beginning therapist) can specify the par-ticular behavior to be changed and, by breaking down the task into a series of successive approximations, can modify the deviant behavior. Progress at each stage can be measured. Said Perkins (1977):

> Because speech therapy is just as behavioral as behavior modification (the former derived pragmatically, the latter from operant learning principles), the same general therapeutic considerations underlie most of the methods for remediating speech. . . . In a word, the clinician must begin where his client can perform without failure and by careful selection of types and schedules of reinforcement, move step by step to the terminal goal. No step is taken until its success is assured. At the first sign of failure, the therapist mounts a strategic retreat to a point at which successful performance can be established. (p. 379)

Behavior modification techniques have been and still are used quite extensively in our field. The principles of behavior modification are relatively easy to teach, and the structure of the approach allays a great deal of anxiety on the part of the therapist. The concrete nature of many of the techniques can be quite seduc-tive to novice therapists. The 1970s, when behavior modification took hold in our field, seemed to be what could be called the "Fruit Loop" decade. One could rarely stick one's head into a therapy observation room without seeing a student clinician reinforcing a child's behavior with a Fruit Loop.

The literature is replete with behavior modification schemes. For example, Shames and Florance (1982) recommended a behavioral approach to shaping fluency in young people who stuttered; Moore (1982) recommended behavioral modification to eliminate or reduce vocal abuse; and Cottrel, Montague, Farb, and Throne (1980) used operant techniques for teaching vocabulary to children with developmental delays. Operant techniques have been used extensively in audiology to condition difficult-to-test populations to respond to sound (Lloyd, Spradlin, & Reid, 1968; Yarnell, 1983).

Among the many studies using the operant approach, two stand out: Stech, Curtiss, Troesch, and Binnie (1973) described the ways in which the *client* conditions and shapes the therapist's behavior. (The client strikes back!) Perhaps the ultimate study in behaviorism in our field, however is Starkweather's (1974) scheme to use earphones to condition the student clinician while the student was conditioning the client. (One wonders who was conditioning the supervisor.)

Limitations

The behavioral approach presupposes a very narrow view of the speech and hearing clinician's role and responsibilities, reducing the clinical task to one of dispensing cereal. The mystery and art of client–clinician relationships are not developed. This approach also leaves unattended the issue of carryover into the client's environment. Behaviorism would predict that a number of reinforcers in the client's environment are maintaining the deviant behavior and that these reinforcers are not addressed by working solely with the client. The behavioral approach is clearly able to modify superficial behavior but does not deal with such nebulous concepts as personal growth, self-esteem, and anxiety because it is hard to specify the overt behaviors of these phenomena. However, these concepts may have considerable effect on communication behavior and may be very useful for accomplishing therapeutic change.

A consequence of the unrealistic use of behaviorism to control behavior may be the loss of altruism. Philosophers and psychologists have postulated that the human species is one that demonstrates altruistic behavior, that is, doing good for the sake of doing good. (Although a strict behaviorist might say we do good because it feels good and we thus get reinforced for altruistic behavior.) Nevertheless, I think behaviorism would encourage a "What's in it for me attitude," which in turn would encourage superficial changes in behavior to conform to the extrinsic reinforcer. It remains to be seen whether a child, for example, can see good speech as something valuable in its own right or as a tedious prerequisite to getting a reward; if it is the latter, there is little likelihood of carryover outside of the therapy room.

It is also clear that we do have choices about our behavior (an idea that behaviorists resist). If the college professor who was conditioned by the class had been made aware of what was happening, he could have resisted the conditioning and lectured from the center of the room, albeit discomforted by the fact that the class appeared to be asleep. (Come to think of it, I have had college teachers who lectured while the class slept.) It is our awareness of what is happening to us and our willingness to assume responsibility for how we behave that will enable us to control environmental reinforcers; these reinforcers may not be as powerful in shaping behavior in humans as they appear to be in laboratory animals.

Humanistic Counseling

Parallel with the development of behaviorism in the United States was the development of humanistic psychology, known as the "third force" (i.e., third after Freudian psychoanalysis and Watsonian behaviorism). The theoretical and clinical underpinnings of the humanistic movement in the United States were provided by Carl Rogers and Abraham Maslow. Maslow (1962) postulated that humans have an innate drive to grow that he called *self-actualization*. This self-actualization drive is very frequently thwarted by teaching and parenting that direct the child to look to others for approval and wisdom. Therefore, the goal of therapy is to help the person remove the barriers to the self-actualizing drive and learn to respond to the realm of inner promptings, where true wisdom lies.

A book written by psychiatrist Sheldon Kopp offered an excellent description of the humanistic therapeutic process. The book has the marvelous title of *If You Meet the Buddha on the Road, Kill Him!* (1972), which comes from an old Buddhist admonition that any Buddha one meets on the road must be a false one because the true Buddha is within oneself. As you can see, the roots of humanism are quite ancient. Lao-tzu, a Chinese sage who wrote 2,500 years ago, articulated the humanistic credo so well when he stated the following:

If I keep from meddling with people, they take care of themselves.
If I keep from commanding people, they behave themselves.
If I keep from preaching at people, they improve themselves.
If I keep from imposing on people, they become themselves.
(Bynner, 1962, p. 32)

The application of humanistic principles to the clinical population is reflected in the monumental works of Carl Rogers. His seminal work, *Client*

Centered Therapy (1951), marked an ideological turning point in contemporary clinical psychology (Arbuckle, 1970). At that time, psychologists were concerned mainly with vocational counseling, intelligence testing, and personality evaluations. The client-centered counseling of Rogers placed little emphasis on diagnosis and testing; instead, it stressed the quality of the interpersonal relationship as the means for promoting client growth. According to Rogers, there are three preconditions for change within a therapeutic environment. First, the counselor must develop an *unconditional regard* for the client so that the client feels free to express anything he or she wishes. This is fostered by nonjudgmental listening and valuing of the client within a relationship that promotes total acceptance. The client is never given a label such as "neurotic," or "mentally retarded" but is always accepted on his or her own terms.

Second, the counselor must practice *empathetic listening*, what Rogers referred to as hearing the "faint knocking." This has also been called "reflective listening" and is the most seemingly teachable of humanistic techniques. Unfortunately, if the technique is practiced without empathy, it will fail miserably, as it usually does in the hands of a novice practitioner who is focused on techniques and not on the client (discussed further in Chapter 6). In empathetic listening, the counselor reflects back to the client the feelings conveyed in the message.

The third condition, and probably the most difficult to achieve, is that of *counselor congruence*. Said Rogers (1980),

> When my experiencing of this moment is present in my awareness and when what is present in my awareness is present in my communication, then each of these three levels matches or is congruent. At such moments I am integrated or whole, I am completely in one piece. Most of the time, I, like everyone else, exhibit some degree of incongruence. I have learned, however, that realness, or genuineness, or congruence—whatever term you wish to give it—is a fundamental basis for the best of communication. (p. 15)

Counselor congruence demands that the counselor be in touch with his or her own needs and experiences. It suggests that a "wholeness" is necessary for the counselor to be completely "there" for the client. Armed with unconditional regard, empathy, and congruence, the counselor enters into a therapeutic alliance with the client so as to release the client's self-actualizing drive. Client-centered therapy assumes that with these facilitative conditions, the client's vast resources for self-understanding and growth will be tapped and change will occur.

Applications to Communication Disorders

Speech–language pathology and audiology have a long humanistic history, going back to some of our earliest practitioners. Backus and Beasley (1951) believed that "speech therapy more and more is shifting away from an orientation based primarily upon devices, toward one based primarily on therapeutic relationships" (p. 2). Cooper (1966) reported that client progress for persons who stuttered was related to the nature of the affect interchange between the client and the clinician. He also noted that important similarities exist between stuttering therapy and psychotherapy. E. Webster (1966, 1977) consistently argued for a humanistic counseling model for the speech–language pathologist/ audiologist, especially in relationship to parents but also in therapeutic encounters. Caracciolo, Rigrodsky, and Morrison (1978) reported on the use of a Rogerian nondirective approach in the supervision of student clinicians. Their hope was that if the supervisor modeled the Rogerian approach to the student clinician, the would-be clinician could transfer this to the client relationship. In the field of communication disorders, probably no one has been as consistently humanistic in both clinical behavior and writing as Albert Murphy (1982), who wrote the following:

> Happiness in the noblest sense comes in large measure through helping relationships with others, stretching our professional resources and the resource of the mind and the heart. Every now and then something in our deeper selves enables us to realize that what truly counts in life is not a matter of what is in you or what is in me but of what occurs between us. That divine spark of relationship may be the most fundamental life force of all. (p. 473)

Limitations

The problem with the humanistic approach is how to apply it to the field of communication disorders. The concepts of congruence, empathy, and self-actualization are nebulous and are not readily amenable to measurement or, for that matter, to the teaching and training of student clinicians. Humanism requires a leap of faith: With the right therapeutic environment, the self-actualizing drive will "bubble" through. Clinicians thus are left in a potentially uncomfortable, unstructured framework. Humanism demands that the clinician yield power to the client to determine the course of therapy—the "lesson plan" is thrown out or, even better, is devised by both the client and the clinician in a spontaneous, egalitarian manner. Humanism places a great deal of responsibility on the client and demands a great deal of self-confidence on the part of the clinician.

Clinicians must learn behavior that appears to be contrary to what is usually thought of as professional. They must listen instead of prescribe. A humanistic approach is very difficult to employ, especially for a young, insecure therapist who doesn't have the experience and confidence necessary to allow for an unstructured, spontaneous interchange with the client. It is also difficult to see how to apply humanistic precepts to difficult clinical populations such as very young children and adults with severe brain damage.

Existentialism

Paralleling the development of humanism in the United States was the development of existential philosophy in Europe. The existentialists emerged on the rediscovery by the French intellectual movement of the work of the mid–19th-century Danish philosopher Søren Kierkegaard (Yalom, 1980). Existential philosophers were attempting to look at the problems of human existence without the comfort provided by traditional religious thought. They were very much a part of the scientific revolution that was then taking place in Europe to a movement that placed a heavy emphasis on distinguishing facts from beliefs. To existentialists, the problems of living are related to the facts of existence, namely, that we must die, that we have freedom, that we are alone, and that life is meaningless.

Existential thought also became the basis of an approach to psychotherapy. Therapists such as Victor Frankl, Erich Fromm, and Rollo May began to use existential philosophy as a basis for understanding and examining the problems presented by their patients. Almost all of the existential therapists were latter-day psychoanalysts. In traditional psychoanalytic thought, anxiety is seen as the motivating force for a patient's deviant behavior. For the traditional Freudian the source of this anxiety is the conflict between the instinctual drives such as Thanatos (death) and Eros (life) or between the Id (the pleasure drive) and the Superego (the social restrictions as incorporated within the infant by the parent in the form of the conscience). According to Freudians, the resultant anxiety from these conflicts is the source of neurotic behavior.

Existential psychotherapy is a dynamic therapy that also postulates anxiety as the motivating force. For the existential psychotherapist, however, anxiety occurs when the individual confronts the facts of existence: death, freedom (which involves responsibility), loneliness, and meaninglessness. Neurotic behavior arises from the avoidance of dealing with the basic issues of existence.

Existentialists do not take a developmental view of behavior in that they are not especially concerned with promoting insight into people's early history in order to understand current behavior. This is contrasted with traditional psychotherapy, which is historically based and seeks to help patients gain insight into their past in order to understand their present behavior.

Existentialism is a very "here and now" therapy that focuses on the present and sees the client's current behavior as reflecting some clash with one of the existential issues. The avoidance of the existential issues is viewed as creating the anxiety that ultimately gets us into interpersonal or intrapersonal difficulties.

Existential Issues

Death

Death, the single most important issue of life, is a topic that most people avoid. Mitford (1963) pointed out how funeral directors increase their profits by catering to our death avoidance—providing elegant clothing for the deceased, a soft and buoyant mattress, and of course the marvelous euphemism of a "slumber room" for the last viewing of the elegant coffin that contains the "sleeping" corpse. Existential philosophers tell us that if we continue with death avoidance, we will live a life of death anxiety—one in which we tend to postpone things and procrastinate without fully appreciating our everyday existence. If we do not recognize the boundaries of our existence, we tend to avoid enjoying the commonplace. (After all, we are going to live forever!) The fear of death is always greatest in those who feel that they have not lived their lives fully. According to Yalom (1989), "A good working formula is the more unlived the life or unrealized potential, the greater the death anxiety" (p. 6).

On the other hand, with death awareness, persons savor and enjoy every moment of the day. They are aware of how transitory and finite life is; they do not squander their time. Yalom (1980) found that the following changes in the lives of patients with cancer occurred when they came to grips with their impending death:

- a rearrangement of life's priorities; a trivializing of the trivial

- a sense of liberation, being able to choose not to do those things that they did not wish to do

- an enhanced sense of living in the immediate present rather than postponing life until retirement or some other part of the future

- a vivid appreciation of the elemental facts of life—the changing seasons, the wind, falling leaves, the last Christmas

- deeper communication with loved ones than before the crisis
- fewer interpersonal fears, less concerns about rejection, greater willingness to take risks than before the crisis. (p. 64)

We are all terminal. How nice it would be if we could all develop and live with an awareness of that fact without having to develop cancer first. Unfortunately, for most people, living with death awareness comes about only as a result of a life crisis.

Responsibility

The existentialists are unyielding on the issue of responsibility; it is the basis of their therapy. To an existential therapist/philosopher, each person is responsible for his or her life and for constituting his or her reality. There is no blame and therefore no guilt—just a clear-eyed statement of the facts. Existence is you doing you! This uncompromising position leaves an individual feeling very uncomfortable because there is no one else to blame for failure. For an existentialist, an individual is making choices at all times, including the choice of how to respond to an event in life. For example, although a person does not choose to be born deaf or to have a stroke, the person does have a choice about how to deal with it. David Wright, a poet and adult who is deaf, has written elegantly about his deafness and about disabilities in general. He found many positives:

> The handicapped are less at the mercy of vague unhappiness that afflicts so many, especially those without aim in life, whose consequent boredom promotes what used to be called spleen. The disabled have been given a built-in, ready-packed objective, which is always present; a definite impediment to get the better of. Like the prospect of hanging, it concentrates the faculties wonderfully (1969, p. 111)

As a counselor, one never feels sorry for a client because the client always has a choice about what to do about the disorder; the responsibility of choice also presents an opportunity to grow. We are defined in life by the choices we make. I think assumption of responsibility is the basis of all change and growth. The first step in all therapeutic change is assuming responsibility. If one feels no responsibility for one's predicament, then how can one change it?

The pathology of responsibility evasion can range from the profound to the commonplace, and we all try more or less to evade responsibility in some way. In his classic book *Escape from Freedom*, Erich Fromm (1941) asserted that on a societal level, freedom engenders anxiety; hence, totalitarian forms of government developed as a protection against the responsibility required to maintain a democracy. There is probably no more common occurrence of responsibility evasion than in the addicted personality of the smoker or the alcoholic. Smoking or drinking is not something that happens to a person; it is something a person does to himself or herself. The smoker or the alcoholic may feel as if he or she *has to* smoke a cigarette or have a drink, but the existential truth of the matter is that the person is choosing to smoke or drink. (There is evidence that alcoholics in particular have a different physiological response to alcohol than nonalcoholics, but this must never be an excuse; it still comes down to choice.) Addicts who will succeed in quitting are the ones who assume responsibility for their own behavior, recognizing that nobody is going to make the change for them. They also need a great deal of emotional support, such as that provided by groups like Alcoholics Anonymous. It is never easy to give up an addiction, but without responsibility assumption, it is impossible. The existentialists are unyielding on this point. One cannot even complain about the weather! I like the Ralph Waldo Emerson quote that "This would be a perfect day if we but knew what to do with it!" So, even with "bad" weather, it is our responsibility to make a good day of it.

Loneliness

Each of us is alone in the universe; after birth, we can no longer merge with anyone else. According to existentialists, almost all of childhood anxiety stems from an awareness of this separation. The infant, who is not capable of surviving on his or her own, cannot bear to be separated from the parents because separation is death. Thus is born the terror of separation and loneliness. Yet we are alone, and that crushing fact is central to existential thought. When we experience and accept our existential loneliness, we find our mature love.

Loneliness anxiety gives rise to romantic love, the kind that is described in song lyrics, the kind that states, "I will die if you leave me." Romantic love fosters a mutually dependent relationship in which there is no growth. Scott Peck (1978), who devoted a considerable portion of his book *The Road Less Traveled* to a discussion of love, sees romantic love as a biological "trap" planned by nature to ensure marriage and the survival of the species. Romantic love may also be an evolutionary step on the way to mature love, which Peck defined as "the will to extend one's self for the purpose of nurturing one's own or another's spiritual growth" (p. 81). All definitions of mature love involve a separation that allows for growth.

The route to mature love may be through a crisis experience that brings us face to face with our existential loneliness. Moustakes (1961), who has written extensively about loneliness and how it relates to love, recounted his experience when he had to make a decision regarding major surgery for his critically ill daughter:

> It was a terrible responsibility, being required to make a life or death decision, for someone else. This awful feeling, this overwhelming sense of responsibility, I could not share with anyone. I felt utterly alone, entirely lost and frightened; my existence was absorbed in the crisis. No one fully understood my terror or how this terror gave impetus to deep feelings of loneliness and isolation, which had been dormant within me. There at the center of my being, loneliness aroused me to a self-awareness I had never known before. (p. 2)

Encountering our loneliness is a means of finding our unconditional regard for humanity. It is a "boundary experience," much like death awareness, which promotes self-growth. The love that stems from our loneliness encounter can be a love that comes from our richness; in the giving of it, we renew ourselves.

Meaninglessness

For the existentialists, there is no extrinsic meaning to the world. For them, we are huddled on this planet hurtling through space in the face of cosmic indifference. The meaninglessness of the universe is central to existential thought in that the discovery of meaning for human beings is that which they construct for themselves. There is no "objective" truth, only a subjective one that is therefore highly individualistic. There is a world out there, but it is given form and substance only by human interpretation. In the face of a meaningless world, we must construct our own vision of the purpose and meaning in life. Thus, one could take a traditional religious view (e.g., "We are here to fulfill God's design"), an altruistic view (e.g., "We are here to do good"), a dedicated view (e.g., "We are here to solve a particular problem"), a humanistic view (e.g., "We are here to self-actualize"), or a hedonistic view (e.g., "We are here to have a good time").

An existential therapist is always seeking to understand the client's particular view of the world. For existential therapists, there is never any judgment of good or bad; it is a matter of understanding what *is* and proceeding from there.

Applications to Communication Disorders

Existential thought has a very wide application to our field. The existential issues abound within all our clinical interactions. Since I discovered the vocabulary and ideas of the existentialists, I have felt the excitement of the Molière character who discovers that he has been speaking prose all his life. Yalom (1980) commented that psychiatrists do not deal with these issues because they have not resolved them for themselves. I think that statement is partly true for me, but I have also needed the theoretical framework in order to see client behavior and to work through many of these issues for myself. Farran, Keane-Hagerty, Salloway, Kupferer, and Wilkin (1991) found existential issues to be abundant in the caregivers of patients with Alzheimer's disease. It was through suffering that many caregivers were able to assume responsibility for themselves and find meaning in their lives. My wife's illness, for example, helped us to live authentically, making everything count, and gave meaning and focus to our life together.

The death issue is always present in our clinical work. In many cases, we are dealing with people who have undergone a traumatic change. All change involves a death in that we must give up and lose something. (We also get something, but we don't always recognize it at the time.) Parents of children who are deaf must give up the dream of having a "normal" child and also of having a "normal" life. The client with aphasia and his or her family may have to give up the person as a viable communicating human being; this is a death. Many of our clients, especially those undergoing laryngectomies or strokes, have literally had near-death experiences. This can leave them very frightened as they realize their vulnerability or mobilized as they realize how little time they have left. M. Webster (1982), a speech–language pathologist who suffered a stroke, found that with recovery "things like trees, flowers, sunsets and friends and loved ones are more appreciated" (p. 237).

Death awareness mobilizes the client and the clinician. When you are aware that death can touch you at any time, you abandon timidity; you want to extract the most from every encounter and you recognize that nothing is permanent. For the clinician, termination is an important clinical tool. All meetings need to have a very definite closure. Group meetings become more intense as the hour for termination draws near. Clients are motivated to work hard when they know that they have a very limited time to be with the clinician. There is experimental support for these ideas. Shlien, Mosak, and Dreikors (1962) found that patients within a time-limited counseling program made more progress than did patients within a counseling program with no imposed time limits. Munro and Bach (1975) found that college students seeking counseling services displayed significantly more gains in self-acceptance and increased independence when they were enrolled in time-limited therapy (eight sessions) than did a control group of students who had no time limitation.

When both clinician and client recognize that there is limited time, the emphasis in therapy becomes one of quality of endeavor. Time per se does not heal; only activity does. However, with an awareness of time limitation comes an increase in activity and an increase in risk.

The freedom/responsibility issue is vital to any therapeutic progress and to any carryover of the behavior into the client's life. In my own observations of many therapeutic relationships, I have often seen clinicians fail to give responsibility for choice and behavior to the client. I often find that there is so much "rescuing" that the clients are not empowered and therefore do not grow. Geri Jewell, an actress with cerebral palsy, felt that the biggest impediment to her growing up was that teachers had low expectations for her and did not require her to assume responsibility ("ASHA Interview," 1983). One sees the problem of low expectations repeatedly in the deaf population. White (1982) reported on a series of workshops he conducted with teachers and counselors at six schools for the deaf. Two hundred eighty-one participants were asked to rank 24 social competencies lacking among the deaf. The social issue ranked first by almost all participants was "taking responsibility for own actions."

Using the language of transactional analysis, Hornyak (1980) pointed out the dangers for speech–language pathologists in rescuing clients—it robs the client of autonomy and keeps him or her feeling powerless. According to Hornyak, in the therapy contact the client should be perceived as a human being who is not helpless.

When professionals become the ultimate rescuers of the people they are helping, they limit growth and keep clients from assuming responsibility for their own behavior. This is referred to in the psychological literature as *learned helplessness*. Somehow we must teach clients who stutter to take responsibility for their nonfluency, clients with voice disorders to take responsibility for their vocal behavior, and clients with phonic disorders to take responsibility for their misarticulations. They must realize that the change comes from inside rather than from external sources. When clients recognize and experience their own powers and responsibilities, they can alter specific speech behavior and maintain changes outside the therapeutic relationship.

The loneliness concept has wide application to our field. To have a communication disorder is to be cut off from contact with others. This is very anxiety provoking. I experience this anxiety every time I am in the deaf community. My sign language skills are very limited, almost nonexistent, despite three beginning sign language courses in which I finally learned how to distinguish *D* from *F*. In the presence of people who are facile with sign language and for whom it is their primary means of communication, I am an individual with a severe handicap. I am frightened, I hope people will not approach, and I seek to leave the situation at the first opportunity. After leaving a group of people who are deaf, I often think how it must be for them to deal with the hearing world on an everyday basis: One could only feel isolated, lonely, and eager to encounter someone with whom to communicate.

As a practicing audiologist, it became apparent to me that the underlying terror of progressive hearing loss experienced by some clients resulted from the feeling of being cut off and isolated. The major means by which we alleviate our interpersonal loneliness is verbal communication; when that is difficult, we become disturbed. The child who would not let his mother out of sight because he could not hear her when she was in a different room in the house, the truck driver who burst into tears because he could not go to the bar with his buddies because he no longer heard the punch line of the jokes they told, and the wife complaining about her husband with a hearing impairment who refused to go out of the house because communication was so difficult for him are, in one form or another, having loneliness experiences. The person who stutters who limits his or her contact with people, the adult with a laryngectomy who refuses to leave his or her home, and the individual with a cleft palate who avoids con-tact with people because his or her speech and appearance are so poor are also very lonely.

Probably the loneliest of all is the adult with brain damage who is locked into a personal "cell" with blocked communication "doors" and "windows." We must break through these obstacles; alleviating a communication disorder is an incredibly tender and beautiful thing to do. There are not many more impor-tant gifts that we can bring to others.

Any catastrophic change in a person's life becomes a loneliness experience because the person is cut off from all of the usual sources of support. Parents and friends seldom understand the person's pain of loss because they are so busy try-ing to make the person "feel better" that they do not respond to the grief; they also feel very awkward and don't know how to approach the individual who has experienced the tragedy.

Suzanne Massie, the mother of Bobby, a hemophiliac, wrote the following:

> The ostracism and isolation were almost harder to adapt to than the dis-ease itself. More than ever we needed the help and comfort of close human contact. We needed friends. In our situation they were essential. I cannot remember a single friend who was near us in the early days of Bobby's ill-ness. . . . It was as though we were living on an island. (Massie & Massie, 1973, p. 148)

The encounter with crisis, as Moustakes (1961) found with his child, in itself puts us in touch with our existential loneliness. How nice it would be to find at that time a helping, empathetic friend who just listens to us.

The existential issue of meaninglessness also emerges full blown from a cri-sis. All of us have a cosmological view—that is, a way of explaining to ourselves how things operate in the world. Most people would like to impose on the uni-verse an order and a rationality that existentialists tell us really do not exist. We need to find a reason for the tragedy, some way to explain it. The most common explanation is that God in heaven punishes the wicked and rewards the good: When something bad befalls us, we feel that we must have been wicked. (This is why in many cultures children with disabilities are hidden: They are believed to represent some "sin" that the parent committed.) The converse of this idea is that God is wicked, which poses a huge dilemma for most people undergoing a crisis in their lives; it involves a very painful reevaluation of their cosmological view. The deeply religious will often say, "This awful thing that has happened is part of God's grand design for me, but because I am only human I cannot perceive the total tapestry of God's intent."

Suzanne Massie, a deeply religious woman, had to wrestle with this big cosmic question of why:

> And yet the need to find meaning remains. . . . Why, God, why?
>
> I could not consider Bobby's hemophilia punishment. When I looked at my bright-eyed child, full of energy and drive, it was unthinkable that God would meaninglessly visit His wrath upon him. . . . Could it be to teach us suffering? The Russians saw in suffering a way to enlightenment. To them it was not a curse but a mystery with great potential for good. "Be glad, Suzanne," Svetlana would say to me. "Be glad you feel deeply." "And remember," she would say, "You are a queen, because you are suffering." In the Soviet Union, a friend told me with respect, "Hemophilia is your family struggle; through it you have been able to glimpse the suffering of our Lord."
>
> In time I came to believe. In time I became grateful that we had been given the chance to see and feel so much. And I told Bobby this, that he had been given suffering earlier than many but that inevitably suffering and failure come to all in life. I told him he was fortunate to have had the chance to meet it when he was young, because those who meet it early are luckier than those whom it comes to later, when it often breaks them. (Massie & Massie, 1973, p. 148)

Vance, who suffered a stroke, found both meaning and agape through her illness. She said,

> But most important of all, I've learned how connected we all are to each other. . . . However, I've learned that my most important work is not what I write about, or what I research but how I relate to others. I am connected to each person on this planet. Some cross my path not at all. Some for a moment only. Some lots of times. But whatever the case, we all are irrevocably connected. My greatest work is to serve and love. (1998, p. 160)

All of our clients, who are cognizant, are constantly struggling with the issue of meaning. Those who are less religious are left with a void that they somehow must fill. Successful families and successful clients, as we shall see later, are those who find some meaning in the tragedies that have befallen them. Therapists must be willing to help clients find their own meaning to resolve the "why me" crisis. This often means participating in or listening to "God talk," an area that is very uncomfortable for most speech and hearing therapists.

The existential issues also have cogency for us as professionals; through death awareness we can restore our zest in our work because any clinician who lives with death awareness cannot be bored. Responsibility assumption leads to our personal and professional growth. Through loneliness we can find the mature love that truly nurtures our clients, and the resolution of meaninglessness gives rise to our commitment; we can choose a path that has "heart."

Limitations

Existential therapy is much more a philosophy than a therapeutic technique, so there is very little for a clinician to grasp in working with clients; it demands that we stay with what we and the client know and can observe. Existentialists are very "now" oriented and seek to explain behavior in terms of the relevant existential issues, but there is no unifying strategy for evoking the issue. Clinicians are left to flounder on their own. An excellent description of the application of existential thought to actual clinical counseling can be found in Yalom's 1989 book, *Love's Executioner*.

Use of existentialism in clinical interactions would exceed the traditional boundaries for most speech pathologists and audiologists. For example, we would find ourselves involved in a great deal of "God talk" with many of our clients. Existentialism demands of us, as individuals and as professionals, a maturity that we may not now possess, but it will possibly be the avenue for our future growth. For me, an awareness of existentialism keeps me focused and grounded in what is important in life and empowers me to make changes.

Cognitive Therapy

The cognitive approach to therapy offers a fourth view of the therapeutic "elephant." The underlying concept of cognitive therapy is that emotional disorder is basically a disorder of thinking. The cognitive therapist helps clients to identify the specific misconceptions and unrealistic expectations in their thinking that underlie their behavior and then forces clients to test the validity of their assumptions against reality. It is a highly confrontational approach in that the client is always challenged to examine the underlying "irrational" assumptions that are reflected in his or her language and behavior. A cognitive therapist is not concerned with the person's past history; he or she is concerned only with the meaning that the client attributes to an event. A cognitive therapist is not directly interested in the emotions—the underlying assumption is that "as you think is how you feel" and if we straighten out your thinking, we will straighten out your feelings. Of the many cognitive therapists, the leading proponent was Albert Ellis, the founder of rational–emotive therapy. He developed a list of the irrational ideas that most of his clients presented to him in one form or another. The following irrational ideas are adapted from his text (Ellis, 1977).

- It is a dire necessity for an adult human to be loved or approved of by virtually every "significant other" in his or her community.

- A person should be thoroughly competent, adequate, and achieving in all possible respects if he or she is to consider himself or herself worthwhile, and he or she is utterly worthless if he or she is incompetent in any way.

- Certain people can be labeled "bad," "wicked," or "villainous," and they deserve severe blame or punishment for their sins.

- It is awful or catastrophic when things are not the way an individual would very much like them to be.

- Human unhappiness is externally caused, and individuals have little or no ability to control their sorrows and disturbances.

- If something is or may be dangerous or fearsome, one should be terribly concerned about it and should keep dwelling on the possibility of its occurrence.

- It is easier to avoid certain life difficulties and self-responsibilities than it is to face them.

- An individual should be dependent on others and needs someone stronger than himself or herself on whom to rely.

- A person's past history is an all-important determinant of his or her present behavior, and because something once strongly affected his or her life, it should continue to do so.

- An individual should become quite upset over other people's problems and disturbances.

- There is invariably a correct, precise, and perfect solution to human problems, and it is catastrophic if this perfect solution is not found.

Applications to Communication Disorders

I think cognitive therapy is a model of counseling that is used a great deal in our field without our recognizing it as such. We use this approach when we set about to persuade clients, as when we list the reasons why someone should get a hearing aid or use an artificial larynx. We are not concerned with the client's feelings, assuming that once the person gets the appliance and sees how well it functions, the feelings will change.

A more systematic application of cognitive therapy has been used for persons with fluency disorders. Maxwell (1982) reported that a majority of his clients displayed a significant reduction in the severity of their stuttering and a marked decline in speech-related stress under a therapeutic regime that employed various self-management and self-monitoring strategies. Emerick (1988) outlined in detail a cognitive approach to be used with adults who stuttered.

I find Ellis's (1977) ideas immensely useful in almost all of my professional and personal contacts. Irrational ideas are reflected in the language people use to describe their problems, for example, the use of the word *can't* when it is really a "choose not to" situation, as in "I can't tell my pediatrician how angry I am" or "I can't use my new speech on the telephone." Translation: "I choose not to." Other language changes that I find valuable are as follows:

- "Should" and "ought" changed to "want to" or "not want to," as in "I should use my new voice" to "I want to (or do not want to) use my new voice."

- "Have to" changed to "want to" or "choose to," as in "I have to stay home and not meet people" to "I want to stay home" or "I choose to stay home."

- "We," "us," "society," and so on changed to "I," as in "We are unhappy with this class" to "I am unhappy with this class (therefore I can do something about it if I choose to)."

- Modified "to be" verbs, as in "I am a dumb person" to "I did a dumb thing and I can still be a smart person."
- "But" changed to "and" (as in all the "yes . . . . but" sentences), as in "I want to speak in public but I am afraid" to "I want to speak in public and I am afraid."

All of these linguistic changes force the person to assume responsibility for his or her behavior and for thinking clearly about that behavior. Underlying rational–emotive therapy, as with all other therapies, is responsibility assumption. I find that when I listen for the irrational assumptions that are reflected in the language of the client, and when I gently change the language, there is often immense benefit to the client.

I find that irrational ideas such as "I must be universally liked" and "A competent and worthwhile person makes no mistakes" are particularly useful in working with both student clinicians and other professionals. People who hold these ideas generally try so hard to be liked that they are unwilling to offend their clients in any way. Thus, students and clinicians tend to meet client expectations rather than their own. The fear of making mistakes severely limits personal and professional growth and seems to be almost epidemic in student populations. I think this is a direct reflection of the poor teaching methods to which our students have been subjected—teaching that does not accept mistakes and incompetence as natural to the learning process. Almost every professional group with which I work is beset by these same issues, and professional growth is usually limited by an unwillingness to assume risk.

Limitations

The rational–emotive therapies were developed for neurotic individuals whose emotions were in significant disparity from objective reality. Clients with communication disorders have very strong emotions, as I shall describe in Chapter 4, and these feelings are based on a reality. It is very normal, very appropriate, and very rational to feel bad because you have a child who is deaf, a husband with aphasia, or a severe hearing loss. My own personal bias is that these feelings need expression and need to be acknowledged in order for counseling to proceed. A strictly cognitive approach cuts short the expression of feelings and moves clients quickly (I think too quickly) into the intellectual realm.

The other limitation of the cognitive therapies is the ever-present likelihood of getting into a persuasion model of counseling. A very fine line exists between cognitive restructuring and persuading. Counselors need to point out "irrationality" without prescribing, which is very difficult to do. By prescribing, one may help to create the dependent client who does not think for him- or her—the reverse of what any good counselor would want. The temptation to get the client to think as we do is very great, but this must be avoided if we are to be truly helpful. When we set out to persuade, we stop listening. We are so busy marshaling our arguments that we do not hear what the client is really saying, and this can be detrimental to client growth.

The Theories Compared

These four views of the therapeutic "elephant" have a good deal of relevance for our field. In theory, the approaches are very divergent; in practice, there are many more similarities than differences. To contrast them, we can use an example of a man going to a counselor to try to give up smoking. A behavioral therapist would devise a plan of cigarette reduction and periodic rewards for meeting the reduction criterion. A client-centered therapist would begin by asking the client what he thought needed to be done in order to give up smoking, and together they might devise a plan. The existential therapist would point out to the client that smoking is something he is choosing to do and perhaps he is now ready to choose something else. The cognitive therapist would direct the client to examine the irrational assumption he is making—that lung cancer and all of the other known negative effects of smoking cannot happen to him.

In practice, latter-day behaviorists recognize the importance of the relationship in promoting growth. Behavioral therapists have come to recognize that one of the first goals of the counselor is to establish a relationship with clients in which they feel free to express themselves to the counselor and in which the counselor is perceived as someone who is interested in attempting to help with the problem. It is also the clients who select the goals of therapy and in concert with the therapist work to change the environmental reinforcers that are maintaining the current self-defeating behaviors (Hansen, Stavis, & Warner, 1977). This view of counseling could be written by any humanist-oriented counselor. By the same token, Yalom (no behaviorist, he) commented that "every form of psychotherapy is a learning process relying in part on operant conditioning" (1975, p. 57). Cognitive therapists and existentialists would agree wholeheartedly on the issue of meaning, and humanists are very much allied with existentialists, although they tend to be a bit more upbeat and less philosophically based than their existential counterparts. All therapists agree that no change can take place without the client assuming responsibility. The particular routes to that goal vary, but many of the therapeutic roads cross one another.

No experimental evidence supports the superiority of any one of these counseling approaches. The variables that need to be controlled to determine scientifically which is a better approach (e.g., counselor competency, purity of counselor theory, level of client maladjustment, and degree and measurement of change) are currently so intangible as to preclude any meaningful research into therapeutic efficacy. We are reduced to selecting a particular approach because it is the most congenial to our personality and our worldview. The client behavior exists, and it is a matter of which therapeutic lens the counselor selects in order to see it.

The general theory that a professional holds about counseling is a reflection of his or her attitudes about people and how they learn, change, and grow. Theory in this context becomes synonymous with point of view, which in turn reflects how the counselor views client behavior. The problem with theory is that it can quickly become dogma and thus severely limit the response of the counselor. I think that we must choose a particular way of approaching clients and then be willing to adapt within the context of the client–clinician relationship. The context will always determine the appropriateness of a response. My own personal view, which will be expounded later, is that all good counseling begins from careful listening and that the client will teach us how to be most helpful. It is our task to provide the client with the environment and materials needed for growth. If we are unwilling or incapable of doing so we must refer the client to someone else.

THE ERIKSON LIFE CYCLE
AND RELATIONSHIPS

Among the pantheon of my personal gurus, Erik Erikson rates highly. The son of a Jewish mother and a Christian father, he also had a Jewish stepfather and came of age in Germany during the rise of Hitler. As a youth he was an itinerant artist, a euphemism for a young man without much direction. He was employed as a tutor in a family that was friendly with Sigmund Freud. Anna Freud, trained as an elementary schoolteacher, was interested in applying psychoanalytic therapy developed by her father to the raising of children, and she became involved with the family that Erikson was tutoring. Erikson was swept up in the psychoanalytic movement and entered psychoanalysis (which was a requirement for anyone seeking to become a psychoanalyst) with Anna Freud. He finished his psychoanalytic training in 1933 and because of the deteriorating conditions in Germany and his Jewish family connections, emigrated with his family to the United States. He worked in Boston for several years as a child analyst, one of the first analysts in the United States to specialize in children.

Erikson subsequently moved to the West Coast, studied the child-raising practices of the Sioux and Yurok tribes, and worked with the children enrolled at the Institute of Child Welfare in California. He became quite interested in how culture shapes personality, and with the eye of a painter and the training of a clinician, he observed the evolution of the life cycle from infancy to death. Among Erikson's many works, probably the most outstanding is his *Childhood and Society* (1950), in which he first delineated his observations of the life cycle. (Readers interested in further investigating the life and work of Erikson are referred to the excellent 1970 biography written by Robert Coles.

Erikson's frequently used and quoted model of the life cycle is an immensely useful way to look at the ego qualities that emerge during critical periods of development from childhood to adulthood. Erikson believed that each successive stage has a special relationship to a basic element of society because the life cycle and our institutions have evolved together. Each stage of ego development or "crisis" needs to be at least partially resolved before one can successfully move on to the next stage. It is possible to think of the stages as a continuum in which the child establishes ego development features. This is a hierarchical structure in which each developmental issue is present in the previous stage and is further worked out in subsequent stages. A stage is presented as a duality, with the usual outcome as a balance between the two extremes. The reader needs to bear in mind that there are no distinct markers between stages and that the process of movement is not a straight line, as implied by the theoretical model. Cognitively, we like to have things nice and clearly delineated; however, nature doesn't always work that way. The process of ego maturation is a sloppy, meandering one that becomes hard to describe and to grasp intellectually.

Erikson's Eight Stages

Stage 1: Trust Versus Mistrust

At this first stage, the infant must come to recognize that the world is basically a safe place—that needs are going to be met and that there is some consistency and order to the world. In order for the child to feel trust, the world must be predictable and the people who inhabit that world (mainly the primary caretaker) must be trustworthy and responsive in predictable and positive ways. It is believed that failure to develop this basic trust leads to the development of the severest forms of infantile schizophrenia.

Stage 2: Autonomy Versus Shame and Doubt

During this stage, the child develops a sense of personal power, of having some control over the world. This begins as some motor control is established and as speech and language develop. The child can make wants known and begin to control others. Unfortunately, autonomy frequently emerges as a negative reaction to the desires of the parents; thus is born the "terrible twos." The child is working on establishing boundaries; the task of the parents is to help him or her develop a sense of autonomy with a benign conscience. If the child is controlled by shame, he or she will tend to become an adult who governs by the letter of the law rather than its spirit and who suffers from compulsive behavior.

Stage 3: Initiative Versus Guilt

In this stage, the child learns to be assertive and to take risks. The normal child moves into the larger adult society in an intrusive manner that is characterized by vigorous movements and occasional aggressiveness (especially toward siblings). An insatiable curiosity manifests itself through the asking of endless questions. The task of the parents is to allow the child to move into the adult world without clamping down so much as to limit initiative. Too many restrictions placed on the child by the parents will cause him or her to develop a highly constricted conscience based on guilt, which limits his or her willingness to take risks. Psychopathology at this stage leads to an adult who exhibits hysterical denial, overconstricts him- or herself to the point of self-obliteration, or develops a great many psychosomatic diseases.

Stage 4: Industry Versus Inferiority

This stage coincides with the so-called latency period, which generally occurs when the child is between the ages of 5 years and 11 years, although when one examines what occurs during this age span, it is clear that the use of the term "latency" is a misnomer. Equipped with a sense of trust in the world and with some trust in self because of being allowed to develop autonomy and initiative, the child is now ready to learn formal skills. Society accommodates by providing the school in its many manifestations; here the technological fundamentals of the society are learned. The child acquires the tools that he or she will need in order to assume adulthood. The danger to the child at this stage is that a sense of adequacy may not develop, either through the failure of the family to prepare the child for school or the failure of the school to capitalize on the child's emerging abilities. An adult who has had difficulty at the industry level develops feelings of inadequacy when he or she compares him- or herself to peers.

Stage 5: Identity Versus Role Confusion

Erikson's recognition of the adolescent experience as predominantly an issue of identity has received a great deal of attention and confirmation from developmental psychologists. The adolescent's task is to establish independence and freedom from the family and then in the latter stages of adolescence to establish a social role. The adolescent uses the parents as his or her first role model, and because the adolescent is also working on establishing independence from the family, he or she will designate the same-sex parent as the "enemy". There is a time when the parents are a total embarrassment to the adolescent. This is especially true for the oldest child; subsequent children have two models from which to work, and they are usually easier for the parents to deal with as they fall somewhere between the extremes presented by the parents and the oldest sibling.

Establishment of identity is a very complex process because it is also heavily influenced by significant adults outside of the family: Other family members, teachers, neighbors, and even characters in plays and movies all influence the adolescent's search for identity. Children raised in single-parent homes must use these outside sources to help them establish identity.

Identity is actually accomplished through life experiences. As we encounter situations in which we have some success and some failure, we get a more rounded picture of ourselves. Identity, thus, is a constantly evolving attribute as we move through the life cycle. Failure to establish an identity during adolescence leads to gender and role confusion.

Stage 6: Intimacy Versus Isolation

Erikson was one of the first child analysts to recognize that the life cycle does not cease at adolescence but continues into adulthood. Adulthood is not static; it is fraught with crises. As a child I often thought that when I was 30 I would "have it all together." I now recognize that growth is a continuous process. At times there are plateaus, and at other times there are "breakup" periods. Perhaps the times when we think we have it all together are just interludes to be enjoyed and savored.

At this stage, the young adult is an independent and self-governing individual; the task is to establish new ties to the world that are free of the family relationships. These ties will evolve into the establishment of new primary relationships and of an occupation. Those adults who have a fragile sense of identity dare not enter into intimate relationships for fear of losing the self, whereas those individuals who have little sense of self try to fuse with another and establish identity through the other person. In a truly intimate, loving relationship, both parties can and do maintain their separate identities. The young adult must find this balance, which is not an easy task.

Work also involves a fusion in which one must try to maintain a separate identity while feeling a part of the institution. An individual with a fragile ego becomes fearful of being swallowed by the institution and fails to commit, whereas an individual with little sense of identity will tend to overcommit and merge personal identity with work identity; neither solution is healthy. The failure to solve the intimacy crisis often leads to a deep sense of isolation and alienation.

Stage 7: Generativity Versus Stagnation

This stage involves the need to ensure the existence of the species either by literally becoming a parent or by sharing knowledge and skills with the young. It is the stage that is characterized by productivity and creativity and an altruism stage wherein adults forego their own personal needs to care for others. Generativity does not necessarily mean becoming a parent. One can figuratively instruct or care for future generations through work or charitable activities. According to Erikson, the mature human needs to instruct and teach. Thus is born the impulse to become a parent, write a book, compose a symphony, and so on.

The mere fact that one becomes a parent does not ensure that one has arrived at generativity. Some parents who have not resolved earlier issues concerning intimacy and identity are not able to give. They are still very self-absorbed and narcissistic, which one would expect to find at an earlier stage of ego development. In a similar vein, one's work can be long and strenuous but not very productive. Generativity enriches the individual as well as society; when such enrichment fails to take place, the individual stagnates.

Stage 8: Ego Integrity Versus Despair

For the aging or older adult who has successfully negotiated the previous seven stages, this is the age of wisdom and detachment. At this point, the individual has the ability to see human problems in their entirety in the face of approaching death. One is able to love on a species-wide basis in the deepest sense. The mature older person continues to grow and to adjust. The mature adult with ego integrity does not fear death and recognizes it as an integral part of the life cycle. Growing old does not guarantee that one will also grow wise. There are elderly adults who fear death, feel that life is now too short for them to engage in any new endeavor, and are mired in despair.

The Life Cycle and Communication Disorders

There has not been extensive use of the Erikson life cycle model in the field of communication disorders. I have found one detailed application of it by Schlessinger and Meadow (1971), who, in their study of deafness and mental health, used the Erikson model as a theory for explaining the discrepancy between "normal" potential and the relatively poor achievement of people who are deaf.

Using their clinical experience, they found the developmental framework provided by the life cycle model to be valuable in looking at the child who is deaf. It appears that at each life cycle stage, children who are deaf have a more formidable task in resolving that particular crisis than do normally hearing children.

One might assume that the development of basic trust may be impaired because of the delays and uncertainties in the diagnosis of deafness and the consequent anxiety of the parents. The occurrence of the parental grief reaction, which involves a great deal of anger and sorrow, also suggests that the child who is deaf may not receive the consistency of parental care and responsiveness that is vital to the development of trust. When the infant who is deaf is undergoing diagnosis, the world must seem a very frightening place involving many strangers and many unexplained parental absences.

A lack of clear communication can limit the development of autonomy and initiative in a child with hearing impairment. For example, the child's parents cannot explain why a rule is imposed, nor can the child ask the necessary questions to find out about the world. Parents also tend to limit their child physically because of the deafness, because they fear that the child may not respond appropriately to danger. There is also high parental guilt, which is reflected in an attitude of "I let something bad happen to you once and I'm not about to let something bad happen to you again." Parents tend to overprotect.

At the competency level, the child with hearing impairment is again limited by poor communication skills and the overprotection of teachers and parents. Much of our skill acquisition is dependent on explanations. Teacher expectations that children with hearing impairments will be low achievers may also limit the competency of the child who is deaf, who also tends to internalize this judgment from significant adults in the world.

Identity problems are particularly acute in the child with hearing impairment who has hearing parents. In addition to the normal struggle to establish self, the child has an apparent choice between the "hearing world" and the "deaf world." The child's problems are compounded if he or she has been raised orally, which too often involves a denial of the deafness and the absence of a hearing-impaired peer group to whom the child can relate or any significant adults who are deaf to use as role models.

Schlessinger and Meadow (1971) observed that schools for the deaf have not properly equipped young people who are deaf for their introduction into the adult world. According to these authors, the young adult person with hearing impairment is not prepared to understand the hearing society's intangible rules and frequently regresses to a more dependent status, much to the chagrin of teachers and parents. It is also hard for these young adults to develop a sense of generativity because of society's discrimination against persons who are deaf. Love and work become very difficult under such conditions.

Almost nothing is known about older persons who are deaf; this is a largely unexplored area of investigation. One might assume that because of the increased difficulty that they experience at each life cycle level, few people with hearing impairment achieve ego integrity, or if they do, they must travel a different route, one that is harder and more circuitous than that of the hearing population.

It would be very interesting to use the Erikson model on other populations with disabilities to see how they are affected. To my knowledge, this has not been done.

The Life Cycle and Relationship Building

I have found the life cycle model to be a very useful way of looking at the development of a healthy counseling relationship, which is critical for growth. At times I can use this model to diagnose relationships that do not seem to be working—to find the point to which I need to return in order to repair the relationship. The life cycle concept helps us to understand how to build a relationship because there seems to be a hierarchical function in relationship building that is similar to the one in the life cycle model: Each stage that is worked on has its origins in previous stages and is worked out further in later stages.

Trust

Trust is the bedrock of a healthy relationship. Unfortunately, many professional relationships are not built on trust, and there can be no growth in relationships unless trust is present. Three elements are basic to building trust: caring, consistency, and credibility.

Caring is conveyed to the client in any number of ways, not the least of which is by active and sensitive listening. Kopp (1978), a psychotherapist, wrote,

> My first task was the creation of an atmosphere of trust within which we can enter into a therapeutic alliance. I begin by listening carefully to what a new patient has to say and to how it is said. I do not yet listen for the underlying dynamics that contribute to the patient's unhappiness. At the beginning, I am only trying to discover how it must feel to be that particular patient. For a while I do little more than try to formulate how the patient feels and to reflect those feelings back to the patient. It is enough

that she finds that I am trying to understand how she experiences her life and that I help her to clarify her feelings without judging them. (p. 81)

Key to the idea of trust building is nonjudgmental listening. If someone is willing to try to hear my fears and my concerns and responds to my feelings without telling me that I "shouldn't feel that way," then I can be more open and trusting. Joysa Post (1983), a speech–language pathologist who had a stroke and developed aphasia, found that the quality she responded to the most in the clinicians with whom she worked was caring. She needed a clinician "who cared and was interested in me as a person" (p. 23).

Trust develops when one believes that people are reliable. Clinicians can demonstrate this quality in very simple ways. For example, I start meetings on time and always end them when we have agreed to end them. If I cannot be at a meeting, I let my clients know ahead of time. If I have misrepresented issues or erred in some way, I apologize and correct the error. I try to be transparent about my feelings and my concerns. I also never tell clients anything that I cannot verify.

In the initial stages of relationship, we clinicians are granted credibility by virtue of our title. Humans often give their trust to someone who bears the title "doctor" (especially if a white coat is worn). Over time, however, credibility has to be earned. In part we as clinicians earn it by what we know and how we convey it. The information given by the professional early in diagnosis is seldom retained by the clients because affect is so high. What is being worked on without either party being aware of it is the establishment of credibility. I will trust a professional if I think he or she knows the field, even if at that point I do not have a sufficient corpus of stored knowledge to evaluate the information being provided.

All the intangibles of credibility establishment are conveyed to others by how I conduct myself, whether I seem to be in control of myself, and whether I share my information. Oddly enough, I have found that I do not lose credibility—in fact I gain it—when I am willing to tell clients that I do not know something. They are then willing to trust the other information that I provide. My willingness to tag something as unknown by me gives them the confidence to believe that what I do say is known. (Of course, there are times when what I think is "known" is not a fact; if too many of these occur, I lose all credibility. It is my professional responsibility to keep current in my information.

One of the surest ways to lose credibility is by reassurance. Although the people we are dealing with frequently seek reassurance, when we give it, we also diminish ourselves. When we tell people that it will be okay in order to help make them feel better, they know that we cannot know that it will be better, and we lose credibility. I am always suspicious of anyone who seems to be telling me what I want to hear. At one level it is soothing; at another, I lose confidence in the person.

Autonomy

Autonomy in a relationship is control that each party has; it is the feeling that I can make things happen that I perceive are in my best interest. Autonomy is always established in relationship to another person; it is a bouncing-off that requires some form of negotiation with that person, who usually is perceived as being more powerful. When the powerful other is the parent, then the child must be given some sense of control—some choices that are respected by the adult. This can save a great deal of grief. I remember walking one time at a fair with my 4-year-old daughter, and it was becoming quite clear we were both getting fatigued. I suggested to her that she sit down; because she was working on autonomy in a big way at that time, her only possible response was "no." My wife, who was standing next to me, turned to her and said, "Alison, which chair are you going to sit on, the red one or the blue one?" Alison promptly sat because she now had some control. She was permitted a choice and her choice was respected. We all need that sense of control in our relationships.

Often the powerful "other" in relationships is the professional. How much autonomy do we allow in therapy? My observation of most therapy is that very little autonomy is granted to the client. I think this is a result of the "lesson plan syndrome." Students in training are expected to enter therapy with specific plans and goals. This gives the therapist, especially the insecure beginning therapist, control of the situation. More experienced therapists will be flexible and are able to modify a plan, depending on the client. How many therapists, I wonder, develop their lesson plans in conjunction with the specific client, where both sit down and decide the agenda for that meeting? Autonomy can be encouraged in such little ways as, for example, the audiologist asking the client after a diagnostic evaluation, "What do you need to know?" rather than delivering a set speech and making all the decisions regarding the kind of information needed.

The professional has difficulty giving autonomy to the client on two counts, the first of which is time. When there is a waiting room full of patients, it is much more expedient to give the set speech and send the client out the door. This expeditious solution is usually the least efficient on a long-term basis, however, because the set speech is rarely retained and the client will generally return with the same lack of knowledge. I tell clients, "I have 15 minutes [or whatever time I do have available]. How would you like to use this time?"

Second, the professional is worried that he or she might not "ask the right question." In the context of a counseling relationship, there are no wrong questions. Generally, if clients do not ask the question, they are not ready to hear the answer, and the information provided is seldom digested. People will learn only what they are ready to learn and absorb. Gratuitous information usually only increases confusion and is rarely helpful. There are times when it is appropriate for us as professionals to provide information without being asked, and when this device is successful, it is generally because we have responded to the unasked question, which first requires sensitive listening.

Initiative

Initiative is an element of relationships that is very closely related to autonomy. Initiative is the positive side of autonomy. Autonomy usually is established by saying "no" in some way in relationship to the powerful other. In some ways it is easier than taking the initiative because the person does not have to take responsibility for his or her behavior. It is much easier to know what is not wanted than to take the responsibility for getting what is wanted. The professional clinician fosters initiative by leaving spaces—teaching by creating vacuums. If I do not take total responsibility for what is going on, then the other person in the relationship has to act. It may seem damaging to my professional ego, but often the less I do, the more the other person learns in the relationship. This means that we are going to have to change some of the definitions of professional responsibility. So often the professional must "do" in order to satisfy the job description and the supervisors, whereas listening and responding are not always seen by either the therapist or the supervisor as being effective professional behavior. We need to change this attitude. Professionals are going to have to learn to be comfortable with silences and with "not doing" so as to create spaces in which the client can take initiative. We grow through the acceptance of responsibility balanced by self-protection. Clients must learn to achieve this balance, and clinicians must help them in this task.

There are some dangers in this approach to fostering initiative. For one, we will violate the client's expectation of what a professional should do. (The client may even ask, "Why am I paying you?") This violation will generate anger, which may or may not surface. The clinician must deal with this anger or the relationship may become distorted. The anger itself can be a marvelous spur to taking initiative on the client's part if the clinician can sensitively handle it. Second, if we do not act, we may lose credibility; there is a fine line that the professional must tread very delicately. The difference for me is in being responsible to (or responsive to) the clients rather than being responsible for them. Although I try to do half of the work and invite the other person to do his or her half, it is often hard to locate the therapeutic equator of responsibility.

Autonomy and initiative as attributes are especially important for parents of children with disabilities to develop. They will need these traits in devising educational plans for their children in conjunction with the public school professionals. It is very easy for most parents to be intimidated by a confrontation with professionals. By now it should also be clear to the reader that initiative and autonomy are locus-of-control issues. Inner locus of control is obtained through the development of initiative and autonomy. (This issue is discussed in more detail in Chapter 6.)

Industry

Industry is the level at which most professionals seem to relate to their clients. There is clearly a task to be accomplished: a communication disorder to be overcome, a child to be educated, a hearing aid to be obtained. Unfortunately, most professionals are so content oriented or problem centered that they ignore the issues of trust, autonomy, and initiative that must be developed first. This professional anxiety over alleviating the disorder gets in the way of establishing the necessary precursors for effective joint work. A therapeutic alliance is not established when the professionals do much more than their 50%, and a frequent result is complaining about a lack of client motivation.

Learning is obtained through any of three routes: by being told (lecture), by seeing (demonstration), and by doing. The most lasting way of learning is the last one. Unfortunately, for parent groups in particular, professionals seem to use the lecture as the primary learning vehicle. Many parent discussion groups are really being run as lectures provided by the professional on some topic that may or may not have been selected by the group members. A lecture is a very inefficient way to teach because it is based on the incorrect assumption that the audience is homogeneous in their knowledge. The degree to which each learner has developed some trust will be reflected in his or her willingness to ask questions and to take some initiative for his or her own learning.

As a teaching device, demonstration is very tricky. If it is not used sensitively, it can "deskill" the learner by increasing his or her feelings of incompetency. I saw this occur in an itinerant therapy program where I worked with both the teachers and the parents of young children with hearing impairment. In this program, the teacher had to travel several hours to get to the parents' home, and she had only a limited amount of time to spend with the child. This teacher often brought in the child's favorite toy and invariably gave a successful lesson. The child was generally very eager to see the teacher because she came only once a week and always brought a new toy, which she used skillfully. The lesson almost always went well, and the therapist would then tell the parent who was observing to continue working on this lesson during the week. However, when the parent tried to do the lesson by imitating what she had seen the therapist do, she usually failed. This failure occurred for a variety of reasons: The child was too familiar with the parent and resented the parent as teacher;

the parent had many emotional issues about the child; and the parent was probably not very competent (why should she be?), which is why she was in the program in the first place. In itinerant programs of this sort, the parent is almost always programmed for failure by the use of therapeutic demonstration and thus begins to feel even more incompetent. My own bias about itinerant programs is that they should be entirely parent centered. I think that the teacher needs to see the parent as the recipient of the teaching and should rarely work directly with the child.

A similar loss of competency can occur when the supervisor demonstrates to the student clinician a more effective way to establish the desired behavior in a client. This demonstration usually is done easily and effortlessly by the supervisor and leaves the student feeling incompetent. The supervisor who then goes to a conference and observes a master clinician at work may also feel incompetent, and so it goes. This is not to say that demonstration does not have a place in teaching—it can be a very valuable tool when there is enough trust in the relationship and when the learner already has established some self esteem.

Doing is by far the most efficient way to learn, especially if one has a sensitive supervisor or teacher observing. Doing requires the highest degree of trust because no one likes to appear incompetent, and by definition the learner is supposed to be incompetent. In order to learn, the student must be willing to reveal areas of ignorance to the teacher. Unfortunately, most educational programs reward competency and penalize ignorance; therefore, students learn to try to please the teacher by guessing what is in the teacher's head and by trying to appear competent when they are not.

Holt (1964) noticed that when given the task of trying to guess a number, elementary-school children would be disturbed by a "no" answer despite the fact that they gained as much information from a "no" answer as they did from a "yes." He concluded that one of the reasons children fail is because they are afraid of failure. No initiative can be taken unless there is a willingness to be wrong. In order for effective learning to take place, we must remove all penalty for failure and we must encourage mistakes (to put that another way, we must encourage learners to take risks). I have learned far more from my mistakes than I have from my successes. The failure tells me where my limit is and where I need to learn more. My successes, while gratifying, reflect skills that I have already mastered and no longer need to learn.

The unconditional regard, and caring that I convey to my learners allows them to take risks. In short, their trust must be present for skills to be taught and learned. Each of these techniques—lecturing, demonstrating, and doing—contributes to learning, and in a particular time and place, each one may be appropriate. As we shall see in Chapter 6, timing is everything.

Identity

Identity is role dependent; that is, how I define myself and how others define me will determine my behavior to a large degree. It is a function of the expectations that I and others have for that particular role. Thus, it is very easy to become role bound.

For example, the role of "parent" has a connotation for someone who is not really involved in the educational or therapeutic process for the child. I remember once waiting outside my child's school to pick her up after an extracurricular activity. The principal, who did not know me, was concerned about a man lurking near the school. He asked me who I was, and I responded, "I am just a parent." Without skipping a beat, he responded, "What do you mean, *just* a parent?" We discussed that issue at length. Parents, as they usually define themselves in relationship to school, are appendages of their child. They provide transportation, supplies, and lunch money and attend PTA meetings to be told things about their child. They are always on the periphery of things and are considered to be only marginally important to the learning process that is taking place in the school.

The role of "patient" also has a connotation of passivity, which is precisely why I have used the word "client" rather than "patient" throughout this text. The whole process of becoming a patient involves losing individuality. A patient goes to the doctor, receives a prescription, and follows it in order to get well. In a hospital setting, the patient is expected to be a very passive part of the process while the professionals do the work. When patients refuse to cooperate—that is, conform to the role expectation—the doctors and nurses are immensely disturbed. Lear's (1980) book *Heartsounds* offers a remarkable view of the patient process from the perspective of the physician. Lear's husband, a physician, found that when he became a heart patient, the attending physicians stopped listening to him and began treating him as a disease rather than as a person. His first act in recovering from his heart attack was to stop wearing the hospital gown in order to retrieve some of his personhood. The holistic health movement, which seems to be gaining more respect these days, puts the patient at the center of the healing process and requires him or her to take some responsibility for the course of therapy. I hope that this trend will continue in medical practice.

Probably the most role-bound individual in the therapeutic process is the professional. He or she usually is defined as the person who has the knowledge and the skill to make the other person "better"; therefore, the professional has the responsibility for making things happen—for being "smart" and having the answers. Professionals are expected to write prescriptions and give advice. The manner of dress is usually very narrowly prescribed (in some settings, it has to be a white coat), and the terms of address are carefully spelled out—usually with a formality that helps maintain a distance between patient and therapist. Most of this self-protective behavior is ingrained at the training level and is readily adopted by the student clinician. A fully defined role is a means of gaining security: If one knows exactly what is expected, then one can conform to those expectations and behave appropriately. The price one pays for this security is a rigidity in behavior that may very well limit growth. In fact, very often the traditional patient–therapist relationship has many features that limit the development of a healthy relationship; in particular, it fails in the responsibility assumption area because the locus of control is external to the patient and in the hands of the therapist. In the wholesome counseling relationship, where there are high levels of trust, both parties are free to take initiative and have retained their autonomy, and role definitions are not rigid, it might be very difficult for the casual observer to determine who is the professional and who is the client.

Intimacy

Intimacy is very much tied to trust. When a high level of trust exists in a relationship, we can risk being open, which in turn leads to a sense of caring and closeness. Intimacy also involves risk: The fear of intimacy often manifests itself in personally distancing behavior, which is often self-defeating.

In a counseling relationship, both parties need to feel that they can say what needs to be said. Only what is important between them is discussed and revealed. I do not have to disclose my bank balance in order to be intimate; however, when appropriate, I do need to relate—either verbally or nonverbally—how I feel about the other person. There is surety in knowing how the other person in a relationship is feeling. Intimacy also involves negative feelings. A great deal of trust is required before I can reveal that I am angry. Professionals who are role bound often feel that they do not have the right to be angry with clients. This attitude severely limits intimacy because true intimacy is not possible unless the full range of feelings that exist in a relationship are expressed.

Intimacy carries with it the possibility of pain. As I become more caring and closer to people, I also leave myself vulnerable to loss when the relationship ends. Because of the anticipated pain of separation, many people limit their closeness. The price of this solution is personal loneliness. Teaching—and by extension, clinical work—is a very painful profession because many of our relationships are clearly limited in duration. The professional's temptation to limit intimacy and pain is therefore very great, which means that we do not develop relationships that have maximum growth possibilities. I have found that when I limit risks, I also limit gains; hence, I have chosen to develop close relationships. The price I pay in June when both students and parents depart is well worth the joy I have experienced during the semester. No relationships are permanent; therefore, I want to and choose to extract the most from each relationship that I have.

Generativity

Generativity becomes the outward manifestation of the skills learned during the industry phase. Now the client can go beyond the therapeutic relationship to demonstrate and develop increased skills in other relationships. This becomes the therapeutic carryover issue.

Out of the successful therapeutic relationship should also come the impulse toward altruism—toward making things better for others. It is no accident that many of our speech–language pathologists were themselves at one time recipients of therapy. Although this might also reflect an identity issue, often it is a reflection of the desire to give back to others something of value that has been received. This is the noblest human drive.

I have watched parents go through the grieving process. They generally tend to progress from concern about themselves to concern about their child and finally to concern about all children with hearing impairment. Parents are potentially a major resource for change, and this desire to help others, if properly channeled by the clinician, can provide huge benefits to the community. Parents can and do become very active in promoting legislation and prodding bureaucrats to do the things that they should be doing, and many stellar programs have resulted from parental initiatives. This very fruitful energy arises from a healthy therapeutic relationship that grows into the generativity or productivity stage.

Integrity

Integrity is the terminal phase of the relationship. Basically, our job as therapists and teachers is to put ourselves out of a job—to no longer be needed. We are not doing our job well if we cannot let go of the clients we are serving, and although this is painful, termination needs to be recognized as a necessary part of the therapeutic cycle.

Because of my own death avoidance issues, I once tried to keep termination discussion in my relationships to an absolute minimum. I came to see that this was a mistake. There is a need to "close up shop," take a detached view of the relationship, and process the experience. I need to bring the relationship to a close, to explain why I did or did not do certain things, to talk about previously concealed feelings, and to express latent feelings of appreciation. I usually feel a sense of sadness and a sense of loss at this time. When I think about the new relationships that will be starting in the fall, I feel a momentary sense of despair at having to start the process over again, of having to go through all the awkward stages of relationship building again. I often tell classes, "Just when you get interesting, you leave." I also wonder if the new relationships will be as satisfying. I also feel excitement at the prospect of encountering new people and learning something more about myself.

Models as Clinical Tools

Models can be very dangerous if taken literally by the unwary reader because they are a simplification of a very complex process. It might seem from reading this chapter that (a) relationship building proceeds smoothly through the eight outlined stages, and (b) if a relationship is stuck, all one has to do to diagnose the trouble is go back to the sticking point. In practice, this is not so simple. At best, relationship building is a sloppy process, with different stages being worked on at different times and not necessarily sequentially. At times, some issues are only partially worked out and then reencountered. Frequently, several stages are being worked on simultaneously. Models become clinically valuable as conceptualizations because they enable us to talk about very complex phenomena by giving us a vocabulary. The reader must always bear in mind that the model is not the event—it is but a particular abstraction of an event.

Clinically speaking, I have found the existential model and the Erikson life cycle model to be particularly helpful. They complement one another nicely. The existential view focuses on current behavior that seems to be universal, whereas the Erikson model gives a developmental perspective within our culture. There are large areas of overlap between them. For example, the Erikson stages of autonomy and initiative are comparable to the existential issue of responsibility assumption, identity and productivity are intricately related to the meaning issue, trust and intimacy are very much part of the loneliness experience, and death of course is part and parcel of the ego integrity stage.

Despite the overlap, these models give us somewhat different views of human beings, and we can use whichever conceptualization seems most appropriate for describing a particular behavior. The reader must always bear in mind that there is no "right" view of human behavior—only a variety of ways to interpret a particular facet of behavior.

CHAPTER

4

THE EMOTIONS OF
COMMUNICATION DISORDERS

To have a communication disorder is also to have strong feelings; this is true for both the client and his or her family. Communication is so basic to humanness that when it is blocked or distorted we become emotionally upset. Often the display of feelings is very distressing to the speech and hearing professional, in part, I think, because of the lack of training in affect counseling. For most professionals in our field, there is an underlying supposition that the people we encounter are so emotionally fragile that any mistake on our part might send them over the edge. This makes us wary of exposing our own feelings and those of our client. When I first began my career as an audiologist, I think I tried to forestall emotional displays because I was embarrassed by them and because I did not know how to react appropriately. I also felt vaguely guilty and that I had somehow caused the pain; and in some ways I had, by being the bearer of bad news.

My difficulty in handling affect with my clients (as well as in my personal life) led me to employ all sorts of strategies to prevent feelings from emerging. I often used my sense of humor as a distraction in an effort to try to make people feel better. Alternatively, as a principal distraction, I provided information to keep people in their cognitive realm and away from the emotional one. I have learned, however, that the goal of counseling is not to make people feel better but to separate feelings from nonproductive behavior. <u>The feelings must always be acknowledged</u>. I also have learned that people have many diverse ways of making themselves feel better, and that I can just allow that to happen; they are not really as fragile as I have assumed.

The underlying principle of affect counseling must be that feelings just are: We never have to be responsible for how we feel but always for how we act. Feelings should never be judged; however, we can judge behavior to see if it is self-enhancing. In any relationship, it is always a mistake to tell people, no matter how nicely we do it, that they shouldn't feel a particular way when we do this. Doing so only helps them to feel guilty about their feelings, as though they should not have them. Probably the least helpful thing to say to anybody is "Don't worry about it" because then they start worrying about their worrying. What we really mean by "Don't worry" or "Don't feel that way" is that "Your expression of feelings is distressing to me, so please stop." It is hard to see how this strategy can ever be helpful to the very people we want to help.

There is deep pain in having a communication disorder, and in many cases we cannot do or say anything that will take the pain away. It needs to be acknowledged for what it is—a very normal reaction to a terrible situation. Behavior, on the other hand, can be judged. We can see whether it is self-enhancing, that is, whether it is accomplishing the goals we would like it to accomplish. If it isn't, we can set about changing it.

This chapter describes the feelings associated with the catastrophic changes in families that are commonly seen by speech and hearing professionals. Behaviors confound the therapist–client relationship if the therapist does not understand the affective source of those behaviors. In my work with diverse populations, I have found that the feelings associated with loss are universal and are not disorder specific. We as humans tend to respond in the same way to catastrophic events in our lives. How emotions are displayed is unique to each individual and to each culture. The content is unique to each disorder, but the grief process is the same; there is always a sense of loss, and I consider myself a grief worker.

Grief

In all change there is a loss. For anyone undergoing catastrophic change, it is the loss of the expected future that is grieved so deeply. For my wife and me, it was the loss of how we envisioned ourselves after the dog died and our children left home. (They all have left now.) Instead of having a very vigorous middle age, with many trips and lots of hiking and running, which we both liked to do, the reality was her disability; we never planned on my wife being in a wheelchair. Whenever we saw a middled-aged couple in the midst of some vigorous pursuit, stinging tears were brought to our eyes. There is always pain for the loss, and it is a pain that never leaves you. A father of a child with hearing impairment who was in one of my counseling groups told me the following:

When you first find out your child is deaf, it hurts like hell. Then it becomes a dull ache that never goes away. The pain of that loss never goes away. It is not our role to take that pain away; our task is to unhook the feelings from unproductive behavior: As one mother of a deaf child said, "I have the same feelings but they no longer control me."

M. Robertson (1999) commented that the audiologist's urge to deal with practical problems of hearing management often leaves the client emotionally bereft. It is the poorly managed grief response, in particular the anger and depression the client transfers to the fact that she or he has to wear a hearing aid, that leads ultimately to a poor result. This is why, according to Robertson, so many hearing aids wind up in drawers.

The process of coming to grips with this loss is much like the response to a death because it is the death of a dream or an expectation. Much of the monumental work of Kubler-Ross (1969), in her astute observations of people who are terminally ill and dying, is applicable to the losses experienced by persons with communication disorders and their families. However, I have found Kubler-Ross's stages of grief—denial, anger, bargaining, depression, and acceptance—a bit overused and too simplistic for a very complex process.

I am always leery of any "stages" concept in the grief process. I think the process is basically amorphous, having fluid boundaries and being cyclical in nature rather than being a straight-line progression, as has been implied in many models of the process. Featherstone (1980), the mother of a child with severe disabilities, described the grief process well when she wrote,

> I am uncomfortable with most stage theories, they carry too heavy a freight of straight line progress; they also suggest an implausible final harmony. The actual progress is not linear and often is bought at a high price in human suffering. In the vocabulary of stages, acceptance becomes a kind of high plateau, once out of reach, now firmly felt underfoot. Gone are the fears and self-reproaches of yesterday and sighs for what might have been. Matter of fact realism guides our effort. Having struggled out of darkness, we will not have to be afraid anymore. . . . Few parents reach an emotional promised land; most have good days and bad days. (p. 232)

Tanner (1980) wrote a comprehensive article on the grief reaction and how this relates to the speech–language pathologist/audiologist. He commented that loss can be both real and symbolic and that grief is not a single reaction but a complex progression involving many emotions and attempts to cope with loss. I find it clinically more profitable to examine the feelings in loss rather than seek the stages of mourning.

Recently I have come across the work of Shapiro (1994), who sees the grief process as a crisis of identity and attachment. I find these concepts very valuable in my clinical work. There is a constant identity issue in coming to grips with the new reality that catastrophic illness imposes. My wife and I, for example, had to accept the fact that we were now a "disability couple" for whom many activities in which we previously indulged were now lost. Letting go of the old identity to accept the new one is the grief process, but it is a process that occurs in fits and starts.

Behaviorally, the bereaved can get stuck in their loss: They cannot see what is there for them in the new identity because they are so busy mourning the old one. I recently came across the following piece, which I sometimes use in parent groups to help facilitate the grief process:

Welcome to Holland

When you're going to have a baby, it's like planning a wonderful vacation trip to Italy. You get a bunch of guide books and make all your plans. The Coliseum . . . the Michelangelo David . . . the gondolas in Venice. You get a book of handy phrases and learn how to say a few words in Italian. It's all very exciting.

Finally, the time comes for your trip. You pack your bags and off you go.

Several hours later, the plane lands. The stewardess comes in and says, "Welcome to Holland."

"Holland?!?" you say. "Holland?? I signed up for Italy! All my life I've dreamed of going to Italy!"

"I'm sorry," she says. "There's been a change and we've landed in Holland."

"But I don't know anything about Holland! I never thought of going to Holland. I have no idea what you do in Holland!"

What's important is that they haven't taken you to a terrible ugly place, full of famine, pestilence and disease. It's just—a *different* place.

So you have to go out and buy a whole new set of guide books . . . you have to learn a whole new language . . . and you'll meet a whole new bunch of people you would never have met otherwise.

Holland. It's slower-paced than Italy, less flashy than Italy . . . but after you've been there for a while, and you've had a chance to catch your breath, you look around and begin to discover that Holland has windmills . . . and Holland has tulips . . . Holland even has Rembrandts.

But everyone you know is busy coming and going from Italy . . . and they're all bragging about what a great time they had there. And for the rest of your life you will say, "Yes, that's where I was supposed to go. That's what I had planned." And the pain of that will never, ever, go away. And you must accept that pain—because the loss of that dream is a very significant loss.

But . . . If you spend your time mourning the fact that you never got to go to Italy, you may never be available to enjoy the very *lovely*, very *special* things about Holland.

—*Emily Perl Kingsley*
(Copyright 1987 by the author. Reprinted with permission.)

So many mourners feel stuck in "Holland"—always bemoaning the fact that they are not in "Italy." The ultimate goal of counseling, as I see it, is to help people recognize what Holland has to offer, and although they may always regret the lost trip to Italy, they can learn to appreciate what they have in Holland. Every once in awhile, on a particularly bad day, Cari would say to me, "I hate it in Holland," and I agreed with her.

It is the expression of grief that frightens many professionals. I know when I ask my counseling class what they most fear in dealing with families concerning the diagnosis, they often respond, "When the parents cry." (The students are often afraid that they might start crying too.) For me, the overt expression of pain is usually a good marker of success. It indicates to me that the parent is not buttressed by denial and has psychologically owned the disorder. It also requires a great deal of strength to cry in public. I find parents who grieve deeply and openly in the initial stages usually do quite well in the later stages. I worry more about those parents who seem to "take it so well."

Feelings of Inadequacy

Anyone faced with a daunting change in life will, to some extent feel overwhelmed by and inadequate to deal with the new challenges posed by the change. Parents of children with disabilities in particular feel overwhelmed because the responsibility is awesome. When parents are told that their child has a disability—a statement usually accompanied by an admonition from some "helping" professionals that "If this child is to succeed, then it is up to the parents"—the normal terror of parenthood is increased fourfold.

A direct concomitant of the feeling of being overwhelmed is the desire to be rescued, which manifests itself in many ways. A frequent fantasy that emerges in parent support groups is "Wouldn't it be nice if someone came and took my child and brought him back when he was 18, all civilized and talking beautifully!" This fantasy is usually presented with a laugh, but it does reflect the underlying insecurity and inadequacy felt by the parents. (This is also the appeal of the residential school—that it will take the responsibility from the parents.)

In one parent group, a father beseeched me to be the "quarterback" of his team. When I declined, he offered me the position of coach, which I also declined. The only role in his personal odyssey that I was willing to accept was that of enthusiastic and knowledgable fan. I told him that I would be in the stands, rooting hard and sharing all my information, but that he would have to select and send in his own plays. When the professional calls the plays, the parents become spectators and assume no responsibility for the outcome. They may either praise or blame the coach, but they are not involved. Spectators seldom grow or learn very much.

Unfortunately, too many professionals in our field are willing to call the plays (e.g, see Dee, 1981, cited in Chapter 1). It is a very difficult trap to avoid. The people whom we are pledged to help are coming to us in a great deal of pain and are feeling inadequate and overwhelmed. They often say, "I'm just a parent; you're the professional." Because we have a great deal of information and compassion, it is tempting to take the responsibility from the parents and rescue them. To do so, however, is ultimately detrimental.

Probably the best example in contemporary literature of the ultimate rescuer is in the story of Annie Sullivan and Helen Keller. Especially as she is depicted in the film *The Miracle Worker*, Annie Sullivan became a role model and a vocational inspiration for many individuals in our profession. A biography written by Lash (1980) offers a more complete story of the Annie Sullivan/Mrs. Keller/Helen Keller triangle. Annie Sullivan had a very deprived childhood. After her mother's death, the 6-year-old Annie and her 4-year-old brother were placed in a home for the indigent by their alcoholic father. Her brother died shortly after being placed in the facility, and Annie literally had nothing while growing up among destitute, elderly people. Because of a visual problem, she was sent to the Perkins School for the Blind in Boston and received her education among an institutionalized blind population. The plea for help from the Kellers arrived as Annie was graduating, and she was sent to Alabama to rescue the family. It is easy to imagine the young Annie Sullivan as a descending angel or, to use a storybook character, Mary Poppins. She must at least have seemed this way to the desperate Kellers, who had an out-of-control deaf–blind child.

There is a scene in the movie that represents a professional climax. Shortly after arriving at the Kellers' home, Annie was to be introduced to her charge at a formal Sunday afternoon dinner. Annie was waiting at the fully laden table with Helen's father and brother. Mrs. Keller entered with Helen, and it was soon apparent that she had no control over the child. Helen was making gruesome noises and totally disrupted the meal by throwing food. The father and brother left in a huff, and Mrs. Keller looked across the table to Annie in total despair.

At this point, Annie had a choice to make: to work with Mrs. Keller and teach her how to manage her child or to rescue Mrs. Keller by taking the child. If Annie had worked with Mrs. Keller, then Annie would not have become famous and would not have received the credit—Mrs. Keller might have! For Annie to have done this, she would have had to have what psychologists call an "inner locus of evaluation"—the ability to pat oneself on the back and let others get the credit. To do this, one has to be a reasonably congruent person. Given her deprived childhood and her very strong need to be needed, it is not unexpected that Annie chose to take Helen to a shack on the property and literally strapped Helen to her at night. Within 2 weeks she emerged with a civilized child who was beginning to communicate—a miracle! Because everyone who has seen the movie knows that Helen turned out to be a truly remarkable deaf–blind person who achieved a great deal despite her disability, it is tempting to conclude that they lived happily ever after.

The Lash biography, however, continues the story. The effect on Mrs. Keller was profound. In a short time, Annie had accomplished more than Mrs. Keller had in the previous 6 years of trying to work with the child on her own. She was profoundly grateful but at the same time more convinced than ever that she was an inadequate mother for such a child. After all, she could not work "miracles" the way Annie could. Mrs. Keller abandoned any further attempts to actively mother Helen and thereafter seemed to be reduced to the role of loving aunt.

Helen and Annie went back to Boston and achieved all the outward manifestations of success, including graduating from Radcliffe College. However, the closely dependent relationship that developed between them, in which Annie had almost all the control, could not work in Helen's best interest (or in Annie's). The goal of teaching, like the goal of parenting, is to encourage the child to be independent. Annie could not do this because she had such a strong need to be needed that had not been fulfilled in her life. In many ways, she needed Helen more than Helen needed her. After Annie's death, Helen went through a succession of paid companions, none of whom satisfied her in the way that Annie did. She never learned how to live independently despite her formidable and remarkable skills.

The Annie Sullivan story is an extreme example of the rescue syndrome. Sometimes the most helpful thing we can do for our clients is to not help or at least to not help in an overt manner. I have often been much more useful to people who left my office saying, "Why did we go there? We knew all of that before we went," than if they had left saying, "What would we ever do without him?" We work in a helping profession; but to be truly helpful, our goal must be to enhance the self-esteem of our clients and their families. Overt assistance, although often appreciated, is also a statement that the recipient is inadequate and needs aid. Very often the overt aid leads to resentment on the recipient's part and also to diminished self-confidence. To nurture effectively is to give help in a sensitive, timely fashion that may not always be seen or appreciated by the recipient. As professionals, we need to remain very much aware of our own needs to be needed and to be able to pat ourselves on the back. Our goal in helping is to create independent people who no longer need help. When we have an independent client, we will have a superior therapeutic outcome.

Anger

Almost anyone experiencing a catastrophic change will experience some anger. The person might not be aware of this anger and might not be able to express it, but it is there nonetheless. Anger has many sources, the predominant one being a violation of expectations. At a very simple level, if you and I have an agreement to meet and you fail to show up, I will be angry. It is a self-righteous anger. All parents have many expectations about their unborn child, most significantly that he or she will be normal. When the child is "defective," the parents are angry because they feel cheated.

Another expectation that is doomed to failure is that the disorder can be cured. Parents find it harder to accept the fact that there is no cure than to accept the fact that the child has a disability. (They say, for example, "We spend so much money to send an astronaut to the moon; why can't we find a cure for cerebral palsy?") The clients also have expectations of the professional and usually expect to be taken care of à la Annie Sullivan. (They saw the movie The Miracle Worker, too.) This expectation may or may not be violated.

The most pervasive, and perhaps most harmful, expectation that clients have is the idealized image of how they should perform. This expectation is fed by a steady stream of television sitcom families who resolve crises easily and with apparent calmness. The clients and their families thus come to believe that they should also be able to manage the change with a minimum of stress and pain. When this is not the case, they feel angry at themselves for being so "incompetent" and "weak." They are not able to see the reality, which is that they are quite normal. This self-directed anger is very harmful, often manifesting itself as depression and low self-esteem.

Dealing with or having a communication disorder causes a loss of some personal freedom, which becomes another source of anger. When disability is present, our life options are narrowed and we get very angry at these restrictions. We have lost control of our lives. For example, in a counseling session a father of a child with hearing impairment told me,

I have been working for several years to get a promotion in my company. I have wanted this very badly, and today I was informed that I have the promotion. If I take it, though, it means that we will have to move to a small town which has no services for the deaf, and my son will have to go to a school for the deaf on a residential basis. My wife and I consider this option terrible. So now if I take the promotion I will screw up my son, and if I don't I will damage my career. I am very angry and frustrated!

This father's anger is very typical, as is the frustration of many mothers who decide to stay home to take care of their children with disabilities and to forego any career advancements. Spouses must also make adjustments in their life plans because of the illness of a husband or wife. For example, the corporate executive who can no longer function at meetings because of his progressive hearing loss will be very angry and resentful. His wife will also be angry at the restrictions in their social life and perhaps at her being relegated to the role of, in the words of one wife, "a hearing ear dog." These are changes that are forced from the outside and over which people have little or no control. A loss of control always involves a great deal of anger.

Another source of anger, which is more like rage, is the parent's or spouse's frustration over his or her inability to make it better for a loved one who is hurting. This feeling of impotence, of powerlessness, was devastating for me as I watched my wife stagger from one place to another, knowing that I was unable to make things better for her. All parents are pledged to make things better for their children; when they cannot, they feel a terrible impotence that manifests itself as rage. Fathers and husbands are more likely to experience this kind of anger because of their assigned role in the family, which traditionally is the protector. Their job is to stand at the gates and slay any dragons that might be assaulting the family. When family members are hurting, the father feels he has failed, and he becomes frustrated and angry. In women, the anger traditionally tends to be turned inward, becoming depression; in men, it usually gets displaced.

There is also a direct relationship between anger and fear that is related to our survival. Anger mobilizes the body for fight or flight whenever our basic security is threatened. We operate at the midbrain level, with our cortex shut off. Boorstein (1996), a psychotherapist, commented that "It is my thesis that with few exceptions, the root of all anger is fear and that psychotherapy is most effective when it focuses on the fears behind the anger rather than the anger itself" (p. 3). Basic security is most often affected in the families of the chronically ill, and as we shall see later, it is often the basis of much conflict. I also think it is important to hear and respond to the fear in our clients and not the anger. This is a difficult thing to do.

I think most professionals in our field recognize at some level that they are dealing with angry people who might lash out at them. Many of the emotional distancing strategies employed—for example, keeping the relationship content based—are designed to keep at bay the eruption of anger. Very often, client anger is displaced onto the professional. Also, because anger is a very difficult emotion in most relationships, and because frequently it is equated with loss of love, most families do not have good strategies for dealing with anger other than to suppress it. It is usually seen as something very threatening to relationships and thus is often displaced onto innocent victims (dogs, cats, professionals) or turned inward to become depression.

When anger is subverted and not allowed to emerge, it poisons relationships. A person who is angry with me and does not tell me frequently operates in subversive ways. For example, the angry client chronically misses appointments, is bothered by minor things such as the decor of the room or the comfort of the chair, and does not fully participate in the therapy. Unless I can tap into that anger and deal with it, the relationship will never be mutually satisfactory. If professionals do not deal well with their own anger, they become poor role models for their clients. Very often, professionals feel that they do not have the right to be angry with clients. How very demeaning this is to clients because it also says, "You don't mean enough to me to provoke anger in me." Professionals will do many of the same things clients do in repressing and displacing their anger, such as acting like a subversive agent, thereby confounding the therapeutic relationship. Unexpressed anger is like a loaded cannon loose on a ship's deck that can go off at any moment and sink the vessel.

The source of much client–professional anger is implicit, unfulfilled expectations. In any relationship that has any degree of intimacy, the parties have expectations of themselves, of each other, and of the relationship. In a healthy relationship, almost all the expectations are made explicit so that if there is a violation of an explicit expectation, it can be dealt with in the course of the relationship. Less healthy relationships, and ultimately less stable ones, have many implicit expectations. These are the expectations we assume the other person is going to fulfill, but we never express them to make them explicit. When these expectations are violated, we get angry; if we have not been explicit about our expectations, we cannot be direct about our anger, either.

For example, a husband may wake up in the morning wanting to have pasta for dinner, but does not bother to tell his wife. (He figures she loves him so much and they have been married so long that he should be able to read his mind.) So he goes off to work, expecting pasta for supper. Because his wife is not always accurate in her mind reading, when he returns home, he gets something else for dinner. Under ordinary circumstances, this meal would be delicious, but the husband gets angry because it is not pasta. (The reader will recognize here the Italy/Holland issue in another guise.) Because he knows that he did not ask for pasta in the morning, the husband knows he does not have a right to complain about the lack of pasta at night; however, it does not stop him from feeling angry. Because he knows, he cannot be overt about the anger because it would not be fair. This, however, does not stop him from conducting a trial of his wife in his head. Because he is the judge, jury, and prosecuting attorney all rolled into one, he finds her guilty of the heinous crime of not being able to read his mind. He then waits for her to do something annoying that under ordinary circumstances he might ignore. If she drops a cup while he is carrying this load of unexpressed anger, he zaps her, and they have a big fight about the broken cup when he is really angry about the pasta. As long as they continue to fight about the cup, their relationship makes no progress. Relationships can stand only so much of this before they crumble from the assaults of misguided conflict. If they can talk about the pasta, then they can renegotiate their marital contract, and their relationship makes progress.

Many professional–client relationships have failed because of implicit, unfulfilled expectations. Many expectations revolve, for example, around responsibility assumptions. The teacher or therapist may assume that the parent will be doing homework with the child, and the parent may assume that schoolwork is the province of the teacher. The undiscussed expectations lead to anger that is seldom expressed directly. The teacher or therapist and the parent need to talk about their mutual expectations, and an explicit contract should be created. Then if there is a failed expectation, the anger can be expressed directly and the contract renegotiated, if necessary.

It is not the implicit expectations per se that are the problem (although it always helps to make explicit that which is implicit and see if there is a match on expectations); it is the unwillingness to be direct about the anger that defeats relationships. Anger can be a very healthy emotion in relationships. Because there is a great deal of caring and energy in anger, it becomes the fuel of change. If clients are angry at me, I examine the anger to see if it is justified. If I have been derelict in my duty, I apologize and make amends, if possible. If we are dealing with a situation in which there has been an implicit expectation that I have failed to meet, the anger then becomes an opportunity to clarify our relationship and make the expectations explicit. If I am dealing with displaced anger, then we can clarify the anger. Very often, parents are angry with their child for having the disability. Because this anger is hard to acknowledge, it is easier for them to be angry at me; I in some sense represent the disorder. I can clarify that they actually are angry at the situation in which they find themselves and not at the child or me. This displaced anger very often can be rechanneled into more useful places, such as working to help other parents and other children trying to live with the disability. Anger can be a very useful source of energy, especially if directed at politicians and bureaucrats who are inadequately funding or managing programs!

There is never any loss in dealing openly and honestly with anger. It is an important change agent. It took me a long time to recognize that anger will not emerge unless there is a high degree of trust and intimacy in a relationship. Only secure people can afford to risk the loss of relationships by displaying anger. Relationships are usually strengthened after anger emerges if there is an acceptance of the feeling and a mutual willingness to explore the sources of the anger. The professional needs to be a secure person to allow client anger to emerge. If the groundwork has been laid in establishing trust, then the relationship can withstand and grow from controversy.

Guilt

I think that next to anger, guilt is the single most pervasive feeling experienced by the families of clients with disabilities. All parents, especially mothers, feel some guilt for a child who has a congenital condition. I think guilt in general is more prevalent in the female population, reflecting the way that girls are acculturated in our society. They are not allowed to feel powerful; rather, they are expected to be compliant and passive. Guilt becomes a power statement: It says that I have had some negative power to influence or cause this bad result. One mother in a parent group once said, "I even feel guilty when it rains." My response was, "Boy, you must be feeling very powerful too." There is also power in worry. My mother-in-law, worrier par excellence, did this all the time. Her implicit statement was that if she worried about an event, she could control it and thus feel some sense of power.

I have found guilt in many spouses of people with a chronic illness. For example, one guilt-ridden wife thought that her husband's Alzheimer's disease was caused by her not monitoring his nutrition carefully enough. There was also the husband who felt that he might have caused his wife's stroke by being involved in a car accident in which his wife hit her head. This was 6 months before the actual stroke, but when a catastrophic event happens, we always look back to find a cause and try to affix blame.

Mothers, in particular, are prone and vulnerable to guilt when their children are involved. Mothers almost invariably take responsibility for causing disorders. Mothers in traditional relationships assume responsibility for the health and education of the family, and their guilt revolves around the failure to protect the family from the disorder. Because the causes of many congenital disorders are unknown, mothers will frequently look back over their pregnancy to find a cause. This incessant search for a cause often reflects the desire to alleviate very uncomfortable guilt feeling. Parents want to be absolved of their guilt and hope to find a cause for which they cannot be held responsible. Unfortunately, many times a cause cannot be determined. If left to their own devices, mothers will examine minutely all the details of their pregnancy and can usually locate a "cause." It is impossible to go 9 months in a pregnancy without something untoward happening; thus is born the "guilty secret." Mothers may, for example, feel that they caused the disability by not taking their vitamins or by taking too many saunas or by smoking or drinking. Although most of these guilty secrets are unfounded and cannot stand up to rational examination, the mother often takes the blame and behaves in ways that are not productive for her or the child.

A trusting, intimate relationship between the mother and the professional must be established so that the parent feels free to discuss "this awful thing" she has done to cause her child's problem. The nonjudgmental, unconditional regard of a humanistic-based relationship can establish the healing environment in which she will reveal the guilty secret; this is when sensitively given information can be helpful. As professionals, we can bestow no greater gift than to relieve a parent of unfounded guilt.

The feeling of guilt can also stem from the client's religious beliefs and experiences. For many clients and their families, the disorder becomes a reflection of their own sins. Many parents, if they can't find something in the pregnancy on which to pin the disorder, will find something in their past life to account for it. Even if they can't recall the sin, God must have, to have given them this child. In this situation, we must be sensitive to the multicultural differences of our clients and their families.

Guilt is a difficult emotion with which to deal. The flip side of guilt is resentment, but unlike anger, resentment is seldom expressed directly; it simmers and sabotages relationships. Relationships that are built around guilt or resentment are not healthy. They usually founder and almost always fail to grow because the parties feel controlled by their guilt. There is always an external locus of control in guilt. Unfortunately, because guilt is a powerful controller of behavior, it often is used to govern children and spouses. Family environments with a high degree of guilt or resentment are not healthy situations for children because the result is simmering resentment. Parents who feel guilt concerning their child usually experience resentment as well. A child will sense the resentment and react negatively to it. Guilt-ridden relationships contain a lot of conflict that is seldom productive, because it is often difficult to get to the guilt and issues causing the resentment remain hidden.

Most parents' behaviors are driven by their guilty feelings, and guilty parents tend to overprotect their children. Their reasoning is that "We let something bad happen to our child once, and we are not about to let anything else happen." These parents do not let their child develop much autonomy or initiative. They seldom let him or her out of their sight and are uncomfortable when they do. The overprotection extends to the therapy situation: The guilt-ridden parents, not very trusting of professionals or of professional competency, question the therapist and frequently seek other opinions. It is very hard to maintain a long-term relationship with a guilt-driven parent.

Guilt feelings also lead to the "super-dedicated" parent who reasons that "I let something bad happen to my child, and now I am going to make it up to him." This parent works very hard at doing lessons with the child and attending all workshops and evening meetings. Teachers invariably exclaim, "I wish we had more parents like them." What is not realized is the high cost that such dedication has on the family structure. The husband–wife relationship is invariably strained because so much energy is put into the parenting that very little is left for the marriage, and the child's siblings are also at risk because they receive diminished attention.

The biggest damage is probably inflicted on the super-dedicated parent and on the child with the disability. Such dedication leaves these parents little or no room to develop any other aspects of their potential, and there is limited life experience outside of being parents of a child with a disability. Although these parents look very good in the preschool years, when their dedication is usually reflected in high-achieving youngsters, they look very bad at that point in the life cycle when their developmental task is to let go of their adolescent child, which they are unable to do. This parent wonders, "If I am not a parent of a child with a disability, who am I?" This type of parent makes it very hard for children to break away which they must do in order to grow. All parents find dealing with adolescents to be very difficult, but if their guilt is unresolved, they find the situation almost impossible.

In counseling, the guilt issue must be dealt with in order for the family to function effectively. I tell parents that I have never yet met a hearing parent who wanted to have a child who is deaf or deliberately set about causing deafness in a child. When the parent actually has been guilty of some dereliction that did cause the deafness, we talk about creating an expiation contract to enable the parent to "pay back" the child or other children without becoming a super-dedicated or overprotective parent. The contract, arrived at after much discussion and thought, usually involves something such as the parent becoming an officer in a parent organization for 1 year. After that, the parent is to consider that he or she has paid his or her dues.

When the guilty secret is based on ignorance, such as thinking that failure to take a vitamin pill caused the deafness, then information can help to alleviate painful feelings. When parents feel neurotic guilt built on feelings of powerlessness and lack of control, anything we do that empowers them will diminish the need for the guilty feelings.

In any event, a major goal of counseling should be to disengage the parent's or spouse's guilty feelings from the nonproductive behavior. People can feel guilty and still behave in a self-enhancing way. A parent once said to me, "You know, I still have all those unpleasant feelings, but they don't control me anymore." She was a highly successful parent.

Feelings of Vulnerability

An existential fact of life is that we are all vulnerable. If we live long enough, something bad will happen to us, and if we don't live long enough, then something bad has already happened. To allay the anxiety caused by this fact of life, we develop a myth of invulnerability. We think bad things can't happen to us— they happen only to other people. To a large extent, we need this myth to function in our daily lives. Without it, we might never get into an airplane or drive a car; we might just spend our time cowering under the covers, and even then, we would not be safe. There is no safety in life. Nobody gets out of it alive.

When something bad does happen to us, such as having a child with a disability, we feel that our cloak of invulnerability has been pierced. We can no longer live within that bubble of denial as we realize how naked and alone we really are and how fragile our existence is. We have lost the pseudo-comfort that the myth of invulnerability provided. This realization is scary, and it may make us timid for a time. Parents undergoing a "crisis of vulnerability" seem very much like guilt-ridden, overprotective parents. A mother whose child was deafened by meningitis told me the following during a counseling session:

> When I took her home from the hospital, I wouldn't let her outside at all, and I wouldn't let any other children come in and play because I was afraid she might get sick again. When I finally did take her with me to the supermarket, I brought along a can of disinfectant and sprayed the shopping cart. For the first year, I lived in complete terror that she might get sick again.

Anxiety generated by awareness of vulnerability, as opposed to anxiety that is generated from unresolved guilt feelings, can be a positive force. When we recognize our vulnerabilities, we can and very often do reorder our priorities. We can live more fully as we recognize the finiteness of our existence. This is the existential issue of death awareness. The mother with the child with meningitis also said the following:

It made you more aware of things, more appreciative. It made me kind of stop and smell the flowers a lot more than I would before. I was always kind of rushing around and hurrying and not stopping as much as I do now. I'm just kind of enjoying everything as much as possible because you just realize, I don't know, maybe your vulnerability. Who knows what is going to happen next, so you might as well enjoy now. I used to think that that could never happen to me . . . but I don't feel that way anymore. Not in a real negative, pessimistic kind of thing, but it's life and you have no control over it, so you might as well appreciate what you have. Make the best of it.

That statement could have been written by any existential philosopher. If we allow parents to go through the grief process and treat them with the loving respect they need, then all sorts of good things can happen to them. They can learn to take each day for the gift that it is, and although their life is not "Italy," they find that "Holland" also has a lot to offer.

Feelings of Confusion

As they go through the learning process, almost all of our clients experience confusion, which is a normal, healthy part of the process of learning. As we attempt to acquire new information that we do not have the experience to evaluate and a vocabulary that is totally unfamiliar to us, we are confused. Resolving the confusion is a learning experience, provided we are given time and repetition. Unfortunately, clients and their families, especially in the early stages of diagnosis, are given much more information than they can use. Professionals often use jargon and assume that after defining a term once or twice, the client has retained the meaning, which is usually not the case. Terms such as *audiogram*, *audiologists*, and *decibel* are rather esoteric and unfamiliar to most people. I have found, for example, that parents of children who are deaf take about a year to understand an audiogram despite the many tests given to their children and the many explanations given by the audiologist. (At that, they are faster than some students in my beginning audiology class.)

Professionals are not the only source of information for clients. When someone has an apparent disability, he or she loses anonymity. The person can hardly walk outside without other people telling him or her their inspirational story and rendering advice. Walking with my wife in a wheelchair, for example, was an adventure. She got "God blessed" right and left, and people offered all kinds of free advice. If we had not been secure in what we knew, this avalanche of well-intended advice and information would have brought us to despair rather than enlightenment. Information overload can be very harmful because the increased confusion leads to increased feelings of inadequacy and anxiety, all of which tend to reduce client self-esteem.

Professionals contribute to client confusion by providing information-based counseling when the client is not ready psychologically to receive it. For me, as an insecure beginning professional, content counseling was the prime distancing strategy. If I focused a relationship on content (which also met both the parents' and my expectations), then I could be in control, and we did not need to tap into the feelings of grief and anger with which I was very uncomfortable. This strategy severely limited the relationship by defining me as the source of knowledge, and it extended the client's confusion and anxiety by providing him or her with too much gratuitous information too early in the grief process.

As professionals, we do have a responsibility to provide information. As a general rule of thumb, however, I do not give clients information unless they ask for it. I generally ask, "What do you need to know?" When I receive a response such as, "I don't even know enough to ask a question!" (which is fairly typical in the early stages), I might respond, "It sounds like you are pretty confused." This is an invitation to talk about the client's feelings. I have seen professionals who are anxious to get things going tell parents who are too confused to ask questions, "Here are some things I think you need to know." This response must be resisted at all costs because it takes away client power and gives the professional too much responsibility. The content questions will emerge as the clients become more comfortable with their new status and are moved a bit further along in the grief process. If we facilitate the process by empathetic listening, the content will emerge.

When clients ask specific content questions, I answer them. I like to think that my answers are free of opinion, but like most professionals in the field, I have strong opinions. The best I can do is to identify them as opinions when talking with the parents. There is a need and a place for content, even in the early stages of relationships; it fulfills an implicit contract between professionals and their clients. In the initial stages, the information functions more to establish credibility than to alleviate ignorance. This must occur in order for us to be truly helpful, but we also must remain sensitive to the relationship as it is being established.

These feelings—grief, anxiety, inadequacy, anger, guilt, vulnerability, and confusion—are turbulent and chaotic feelings that clients and their families experience when they encounter a disability in themselves or a family member.

These people are emotionally upset and very appropriately so. As was said at the beginning of this chapter, feelings are neither good nor bad, and it is not our responsibility to make our clients feel better. We can, by our calm acceptance of their feelings and our willingness to allow affect to be part of the client–professional relationship, prevent the development of secondary negative feelings. For example, we can help prevent clients from feeling guilty about their guilt feelings. When we do this, their coping process can begin. If we have a sensitive appreciation of the grief process, we can help the client transform his or her chaotic feelings into positive behavior. As a result, grief can become a sadness that enables the client to appreciate what he or she has, the anger can become the energy to make change, the guilt can become the commitment, the recognition of vulnerability can become the means for reordering priorities, and the resolution of confusion can become the motivation for learning.

The Professional's Feelings

The feelings described in this chapter in relation to clients also characterize the professional's reactions. Nothing is abnormal or unhealthy about any of the feelings described. Under the skin, we are all brothers and sisters. Audiologists, for example, often feel overwhelmed by and inadequate to cope with the responsibility of determining a child's hearing loss and of properly guiding the family. This is especially true for the beginning audiologist, who is still developing good test techniques and learning appropriate counseling strategies. Even veteran audiologists experience an anxiety almost akin to panic when presented with a child who promises to be difficult to test and a family that appears hard to counsel. Has any professional not felt the fear of that icy finger of failure? This anxiety can become the spur for continued professional improvement.

Professionals also experience anger. They feel anger at parents for not following through on a recommended course of action; they feel rage, frustration, and sometimes despair when they can't make things better for the child or family with whom they are involved. They may feel intense anger at other professionals who insensitively or inappropriately treat the family: the pediatrician who fails to refer or the classroom teacher who doesn't understand the child's language difficulty. This anger provides the energy that can be used to educate other professionals and make programmatic changes. If repressed, it leads to depression and burnout.

Guilt is also a part of the professional's experience. I know of no responsible and competent speech and hearing professional who suffers no regrets about the handling of past cases. Mistakes—an inevitable part of the experience of all professionals—are our "nuggets of gold." They indicate to us what we need to learn next. All responsible professionals should be operating on their "fringes of incompetence." They should be taking risks and occasionally making mistakes, or they are not growing. Many speech and hearing professionals are needlessly burdened by the guilt associated with their errors. Fortunately, we are not brain surgeons. Almost all of my clients have survived my mistakes quite well. Some have even flourished, and so have I. It is only a mistake if we do it twice. I like the prayer that Carl Rogers says before he meets a client: "Please let me be sufficient." That will have to do for all of us.

Those of us who work clinically, especially in hospital settings, are constantly confronted with people who have severe disorders. We are not given the luxury that most people have of retaining our myth of invulnerability. Daily we meet people like us who are in deep pain, and we often say, "There but for the grace of God go I." The recognition of our personal vulnerability can lead to our being very caring, thoughtful clinicians, and it can spill over into our personal lives, where we can reorder our priorities, much as our clients do when they realize what is really important in life.

Frequently when the feelings surrounding communication disorders are described, the negative and painful emotions are emphasized, while the positive feelings and experiences are seldom discussed. Often overlooked are the marvelous opportunities for joy and growth. Many parents come through the experience of having a child with a hearing impairment with a clearer sense of themselves and of their priorities than they had before their child was diagnosed. Many parents discover that their child's disorder has given their lives meaning and direction. The joy stems from actively participating in their child's growth; they take nothing for granted. When their child reaches a milestone, they rejoice in the knowledge that they helped in the accomplishment.

The speech and hearing professional also experiences joy in working with the families of clients. In the initial stages of diagnosis, everything appears bleak and hopeless to family members, and the speech–language pathologist or audiologist often becomes their lifeline. My most meaningful clinical experiences have been in the intimate relationships that I have had with parents of children who have just been diagnosed as having a hearing impairment. It is very gratifying to witness and participate actively in the grief process. I often tell parents that I will share some of their pain if they will share some of their joy with me as well. I also frequently tell parents that this child comes to them bearing a gift. It is buried under a great deal of hard work and pain, but it is a gift nonetheless. My hope is that within our work together they will be able to uncover the gift.

The Coping Process

Definition of Coping

My dictionary defines coping as "contending successfully with." All coping involves a stressful interaction between a person and the environment. Coping is any response to a difficult life situation that avoids or prevents distress. Successful coping always involves the possibility of growth and always demands change. The people who experience discomfort will grow because they are forced to derive a new set of responses to contend with a changing set of internal or external demands. I always tell every class I teach that I am successful if I make you unhappy. Our clients come with a built in teacher—their disorder. We tend to give to life what life demands of us, and when we are stressed by an external force, we must find within us the strength and the resources to cope successfully. Coping is a dynamic process; it is not a stage finally won and held forever. At times it is a moment-to-moment proposition.

The Four Stages of the Coping Process

Recently, in my research on chronic illness, I came across a coping process model that I have found very helpful in many of my clinical interactions. I want to stress that the model is useful only as a guide, and the stages are not firmly fixed points as in climbing a mountain—once gained never lost—but rather a fluid series of points in which even successfully coping individuals return to earlier stages. Matson and Brooks (1977), in their interviews with patients who had multiple sclerosis, found four stages to the coping process: denial, resistance, affirmation, and integration. I want to look at these stages in relation to communication disorders.

Denial

Probably no single factor impairs client–professional relationships as much as the denial mechanism. Denial must be seen by the professional for what it is, a coping strategy based on feelings of inadequacy. When a person is in denial, there is no psychological "owning" of the problem. The person may admit that the problem exists, but he or she is not engaged emotionally. Denial is a very normal, very human reaction that occurs in all of us.

When I am driving my car, for example, and the engine begins to sound strange, I respond by turning on the radio. If the engine noises get louder, I increase the volume. Although I know cognitively that turning on the radio is not going to solve my problem, at that time, psychologically, it is the only thing

I can do. In short, I try to deny the existence of the problem, hoping that it will go away by itself. My need to adopt this "radio strategy" is based on my lack of confidence in my ability to repair engines. I feel very inadequate around mechanical things, certainly anything as complicated as a car engine. If you were to admonish me about how silly I am to respond by turning on the radio, I would grin sheepishly and agree with you. At this point I use a passive-aggressive strategy that I learned as a child in how to deal with authority figures—that is, I agree with you and proceed to do what I was doing when you are not around. Unless I am given other ways of coping and gain some confidence in myself, I cannot afford to give up denial. If, for example, I successfully completed a course in engine maintenance with your help, then I might hear the slightest noise and pull the car to the side of the road because I feel I have some chance of solving the problem. I would therefore cope with the crisis in a more responsible way than by denying its existence.

Parents of a child with a disability begin to experience feelings of denial any time there is a new demand on parental resources that requires them to be wise or strong. The most obvious time is at diagnosis: Often the delay in getting a child diagnosed is because the parents cannot admit to themselves that something may be wrong. Others in the parents' environment, especially grandparents, also practice denial, and sometimes this happens to other professionals such as the family pediatrician.

Denial persists even when the parents freely acknowledge that they have a child with a disability. In coping with deafness, denial occurs around anything that objectifies the deafness. The hearing aid, for example, becomes a powerful reminder of deafness. Parents may hate to see it on their child even though they know it helps. When they take pictures of the child, they remove the hearing aid. This, by the way, becomes a good measure of where the parents are on the coping model. Parents who are in the affirmation or integration stages insist that the hearing aid be worn for pictures, whereas those who are in the denial or resistance stages remove it. If the parents are in a total communication program, their denial can become focused on the signing; thus, we have parents who never attend class or, when they do, cannot seem to learn how to sign.

The child-centered professional views parental denial as an impediment to the child's progress and gets angry at the parents. The professional who is direct about anger gives parents an admonitory lecture about how important it is for the child to wear the hearing aid or how necessary it is for the parents to attend signing class. The parents agree with the professional; they knew how important it was before the professional told them, but because they have no other coping strategy—much as I didn't with my car—they fall back on denial. Their behavior then becomes passive-aggressive. After an initial period of attendance at classes or increased hearing-aid use, they often revert to denial, which provokes another round of professional ire. If not stopped, this negative parent–professional interaction can escalate to the point where there is no communication between them, to the detriment of the child.

The professional must learn to recognize denial as a plea for help and not as a dereliction of duty on the parents' part. No parents, at least those whom I have met, want to do badly by their child, but their many fears get in the way of their operating constructively. The basis of denial is fear and ignorance abetted by low self-esteem. People cannot be urged out of denial. They give it up when they feel confident that they can be more successful with some other strategy. In general, it is best not to undermine the denial mechanism directly unless one has something better to offer in its stead. Giving up denial—the only way the clients feel that they can currently cope with the situation—without offering a replacement would be overwhelming. The parents feel as if their psychological survival depends on denial, and in some respects it does. Denial thus is not easily given up. By listening and by indirect teaching, which does not diminish clients' feelings of competency, counselors can provide clients with more fruitful coping strategies than denial.

If the professional is focused on the child and is anxious about the child's welfare, parental denial might provoke an adversarial relationship between the professional and the parents that can destroy any productive counseling relationship. Professionals often try to "save" the child from the parents. Short of removing the child from the home, this cannot be done. Children cannot be saved from their parents; all of us, in some sense, are victims of our parents' failings. The professional must not let parental denial impair the development of a healthy relationship. I don't think any successful counseling can take place unless the professional has some understanding of the denial mechanism.

The identification of behavior as denial can be very tricky. It is not always clear when the clients are denying or when there is a legitimate difference of opinion between the client and the professional. Labeling can be used to try to substitute professional "truth" for parental "truth"—and room must be allowed for a difference of opinion.

One person's denial may be another person's optimism. Frequently, when the professional has a very pessimistic prognosis for a child, the parent keeps saying, "He will make it." Children have a way of meeting expectations, and when the expectations are negative, children seldom perform well. I have often seen the parents proved right; there is never any need to diminish parental optimism as long as their behavior is consistent with accepted management practices. This optimism frequently gets translated into hope, and many parents have the "Maybe someday they will find a cure" dream. This dream, which enables them to work vigorously in the present and sustains them when they despair, should never be doused by the professional. There is probably no crueler act than to deprive the parents of it.

There is also much that is positive about denial. In 1962, the U.S. government declared Spanish-American War veterans, of which there were only several hundred in the United States, to be totally disabled. This declaration, which entitled them to receive full benefits through the Veterans' Administration, occasioned the launching of a large-scale study of older men. These men were in their 80s at the time, and the study involved gathering data on all aspects of their lives. I was involved in studying their hearing. As part of the examination, I interviewed them about how well they thought they could hear. This part of the research protocol became meaningless, as every one of them felt he could hear fine, despite the fact that in many instances I had to shout to be heard. I spoke to the project psychologist about this phenomenon, and he said it was pervasive throughout the study. These men persistently denied any infirmity, and he concluded—only partially tongue in cheek—that perhaps one of the major secrets of living to a ripe old age is to assiduously practice denial.

Resistance

Denial blends into resistance and at times is indistinguishable from it. In the resistance stage, the client and the family say, "We have a problem here, but we are going to be a special case. We will somehow prevail over the disorder." Parents of a child who is deaf, for instance, will say, "I know he [or she] is deaf, but he [or she] is going to be a super deaf person. He [or she] will have normal speech, be a marvelous lipreader, and have an amazing job that few people will ever expect a deaf person to have." Shortly after being diagnosed as having multiple sclerosis, my wife ran a 10-K race as though to defiantly say, "Being a cripple won't happen to me." As I watched her stagger across the finish line, I was filled with both admiration and anxiety for her. It was the last race she ever ran.

Resistance differs from denial in that the persons acknowledge to themselves that they have a problem, and they work very hard to defeat it. In resistance, there is almost always a private pledge to conquer the disorder and a rejection of help from any organizations that deal with the disorder. During the resistance stage, clients are unwilling to join any support groups or receive help in the form of meeting with peer counselors. They are in effect a person with a "closet" disability. For example, in the early stages of her diagnosis, my wife and I did not want to meet anyone who had multiple sclerosis, and I found it very hard, if not impossible, to go to meetings where there were adults who were severely disabled by the condition. I just didn't want to be reminded of my potential future. (My wife was much better at this than I was.)

In resistance, a great deal of energy is directed almost frantically and secretly at proving that the professionals are "wrong." Both denial and resistance are used to forestall or minimize the pain of the grief process. In denial, one says, "I don't really have this problem." In resistance, the person says, "I will lick this problem."

The difficulty for clients and their families comes when they realize that they have a disorder that they cannot defeat. For parents of a child with hearing impairment, this sometimes happens as late as the child's adolescence, when they realize that he or she is not going to be the "super-deaf" adult they had expected; another dream dies and the grief process starts anew.

Clients often need to hit an emotional bottom in order to move on with the coping process. They need to see for themselves that denial does not work and that frantic resistance is not productive before they can mourn their loss and move into the affirmation stage. They need to have some confidence in their own ability to cope with the disorder in a proactive manner.

Affirmation

In the affirmation stage, the loss is acknowledged both to self and to the world at large. Affirmation is a statement that "I am now a different person and our family is also different." During this stage of coping, the family is consumed by the disorder, and energy is devoted toward ameliorating its effects. In this stage, families become very active in organizations designed to educate their members and the public at large. One such group, SHHH (Self Help for the Hard of Hearing), is designed as a support and educational group for the hard-of-hearing. In groups such as SHHH, members get an opportunity to establish their new identity as "persons who are hard-of-hearing"; they have come out of the disability closet. This new identity may be taken on tentatively or proudly (as we have seen in the deaf community), but it is a public acknowledgment. In this stage, an intense desire to help others arises. One parent of a child who is deaf told me, "When you first find out your child is deaf, you feel badly for yourself. After a while you feel badly for your child. Now I feel badly for all deaf children." This movement outside of one's own pain is very healthy and marks the transition into integration.

Integration

Integration (also known as acceptance) is characterized by putting the disorder into a life perspective. The client and family learn to live with the disorder and to spend time and energy on other matters. The client is able to say, "I am more than a walking hearing disorder; I am a person who does not hear well, but many other aspects of my life need to be developed." In the integration/acceptance stage, although there is still pain concerning the loss, and at times grief, the changes caused by the disorder are integrated into a new lifestyle with different values. The affirmation and acceptance stages are reached when the individual realizes that "beating" the disorder is not always a matter of reaching normalcy but rather the ability to live life to the fullest in the face of the disorder.

Individuals vary as to the degree and speed with which they can get to integration. Some families appear to be forever stuck in denial, which seems to them to be the only possible coping strategy; they are paralyzed in their fear. Others move through the process very rapidly, seeming to skip stages. The key is self-confidence. When family members feel secure in their abilities to cope, it becomes easier to assume the psychological risk of giving up the pseudocomfort of denial and resistance to assume the responsibilities demanded by the affirmation and integration stages of the coping process.

Coping Strategies

Pearlin and Schooler (1978), in a definitive article on coping, outlined four strategies that individuals use to cope with very difficult situations: flight, modification, reframing, and stress reduction.

Flight

The first and perhaps primary coping strategy is flight. When confronted with a difficult and potentially stressful situation, each person must decide whether to fight or take flight. In some situations, a person feels ill-equipped to cope and that his or her own personal or psychological survival depends on removal from the situation. This may not be the reality of the situation, but as long as people feel that they cannot cope successfully, then flight will occur. The person's perception of events is critical.

Many divorces occur in families where there are children with disabilities, and estrangements seem to occur in families where there are adults with disabilities. Sometimes an adult child leaves a parent to struggle alone with a spouse with a disability. As a coping strategy, flight always leaves the person vulnerable to guilt and loss of self-esteem. It is tempting to blame the fleeing family member, but this is seldom productive. Flight is a crisis of self-confidence, and in my experience, the identified patient usually winds up in better shape after caregiver flight because she of he has found a more stable support system.

In addition to the actual flight, as in a divorce, there is the psychological flight that occurs frequently in parents and spouses of family members with disabilities. This psychological flight often takes the form of a fantasy about the death of the child or spouse. This is a deep-seated "wish" that is difficult for many parents or spouses to admit because they feel guilty about having such feelings. When they do admit these fantasies to a professional, usually there is a high degree of trust in the relationship, and they expect the professional to accept their statement at face value. It is critical that the professional accepts this admission in a matter-of-fact manner. These feelings are very common. I often tell parents and spouses that I don't think they are wishing their child or spouse dead, but that they are wishing this situation, which is so stressful to them, would go away.

Death fantasies may be helpful in preparing for the actual death of a spouse. This anticipatory mourning is seen frequently in spouses of clients with aphasia and in families in which someone has traumatic head injuries. Anticipatory mourning, which helps the person make the adjustment to living without the person with a disability, is part of the psychologically protective transition process that eases the way into an anticipated new status. The person is trying on the new role, which is very helpful, although it generally causes the person to feel a great deal of guilt. Professionals must never judge these fantasies, which almost always serve a useful psychological function as long as they remain fantasies.

Modification

If a person decides to stay with the family member with a disability, then the next strategy that should be employed is modifying the situation. Stress can be reduced by direct intervention that reduces or modifies the disability. The client who gets a hearing aid and the patient with aphasia who gets a wheelchair and language therapy may reduce the stress caused by their losses. All therapy administered by a speech and hearing clinician is designed to reduce stress and help clients and their families cope better with communication situations.

Unfortunately, in our field there are many situations in which the stress of a disorder can be modified but not eliminated. For example, even with the best amplification, many clients will still have a significant hearing loss. We must help these clients to accept their limitations and to recognize that they cannot further modify their environment. The trick in modification is to know what can be modified, do it, and then learn to accept what cannot be changed, which is not always easy to do.

Reframing

Because the cognitive process always determines the emotional intensity of any event, for those elements of a situation that cannot be modified, stress can be reduced by changing the way a person views the situation. This is known as "reframing" or "cognitively neutralizing" the stressor. The most commonly used cognitive neutralizer is the phrase, "It could be worse," whereupon parents or spouses proceed to mention someone in some place who is in more difficulty than they are. This is known as a positive comparison. The problem with using positive comparisons as a reframing strategy is that there are still times when the client or family member feels upset about the disability. When this happens, the individual usually feels guilty because he or she has forfeited the right to grieve. I think positive comparisons may buy some short-term relief but seldom work for long. The disability will always intrude, and the effectiveness of looking for someone worse off begins to quickly fade. There are other more fruitful ways to reframe, which I will discuss in Chapter 6. My wife's response to "It could be worse," was to say, "Yes, and it could be better too!"

Stress Reduction

The fourth strategy is to deal directly with the stress. No matter how successful modification and reframing may be, many clients will still experience stress with which they must learn to live. Each individual must find his or her own individual stress reducers, and what is effective for one person may not work for another. In my interviews with the spouses of patients with chronic illness, I found exercise and work to be almost universal stress reducers. Exercise is effective in part because it is a time-out experience that gets the nondisabled spouse away from the spouse with a disability. It also is an emotionally calming activity. Repetitive exercise, such as jogging, swimming, or bicycling, seems to put the mind into a meditative state. Work serves as a distraction. Spouses can immerse themselves in problems that have solutions and are controllable. They also have contact with other adults with whom they can talk and think about something other than their spouse with the disability. In fact, one of my definitions of a "shadow spouse" is someone who looks forward to going to work and dreads coming home.

Conclusion

When speech and hearing professionals encounter clients, the traumatic events have already happened and the grief and coping processes are already under way. By virtue of the way we interact with clients and their families, we can facilitate or retard the coping process. This is especially true at the diagnostic evaluation, which is usually close to the time of the catastrophic event, when clients' feelings are fluid and apparent; because the impact of the disorder has not yet settled in, we can alter dramatically the course of the coping and the habilitation of the client. The next chapter examines the diagnostic process with an eye to best facilitating client's acceptance and coping.

COUNSELING AND
THE DIAGNOSTIC PROCESS

The diagnostic interaction is critical for determining the course of the client–professional relationship. It is the first step of a long journey for many clients, and it is an imprinting process that sets up in the client's mind future expectations of professional behavior. If the initial client–professional interaction has a feeling component and if clients are empowered at the beginning, then they will expect and perhaps demand empowerment and affect in future contacts with professionals. Unfortunately, because of the prevalence of the medical model, the professional's role is usually restricted to providing information and prescribing what the client should do. In this model, the client is encouraged to become a passive participant in the habilitation program by simply "following the doctor's orders."

Institution-Centered Diagnosis

In the medical model, a professional takes a careful case history and gives tests to a client. If a child is being tested, he or she is separated from the parents while the professional administers the tests. (If the parent is allowed to be present, it is usually as a passive observer.) After the testing, the professional "counsels" the parents by giving the results of the tests and recommending what the parents should do next. As a beginning audiologist, I found the medical model very helpful. I soon developed some set speeches that I could give after testing a child. They were "tapes" I could plug in to describe how hearing aids worked, explain audiograms, and, for parents of children who had been newly diagnosed as deaf, provide a list of schools for the deaf in the area and describe the various educational methodologies used in those schools. On the surface, the medical model seems efficient. Because I could control the interaction, I could block out a prescribed time and see the maximum number of cases in a given day. I could fit each speech into a 10- or 15-minute period and then send the parents on their way, feeling that I had fulfilled my clinical obligation, and perhaps as important, I could see my next patient on time. I also succeeded in limiting the affective exchange so that I did not have to deal with feelings, about which I felt very insecure. After a while I stopped "seeing" patients; the visits simply became routine and mechanical for me.

A variation of the individual medical model is the diagnosis-by-committee process, which on the surface is even more efficient. Many hospitals and educational programs operate this way when they have, for example, an Individualized Educational Program (IEP). In this model, the child is tested by an array of professionals, usually on the same day but sometimes spread over 2 or 3 days. Parents are then invited to a conference at which each professional delivers his or her report. Professionals in these meetings seldom talk directly to the parents: They are so busy trying to impress everyone else with their competency that they are speaking to impress rather than express and jargon abounds. Parents are glassy-eyed and generally traumatized by the whole experience. Imagine the experience from the parents' perspective: having a group of "experts" sitting around a table telling you what is wrong with your child. It has to be a nightmare! The same must be true for the adult undergoing the "exit" interview.

At Emerson College, research is under way in which parents who have undergone the diagnosis-by-committee process are interviewed. They reported that they retained almost none of the material presented to them. They also noted feeling scared and numb. We have yet to find any parents who liked or appreciated the experience. At best, they found it helpful "because they didn't have to make so many trips to the hospital." All found it psychologically painful.

My personal opinion is that diagnosis by committee should be banned by the Geneva Convention as cruel and unusual punishment. It is used because it seems efficient to have the diagnosis completed in one meeting. The efficiency is only illusory; diagnosis by committee is convenient for the institution or the professionals but it is not efficient when one examines its effects on the families. Instead of retaining what is said, family members remember unimportant details such as the color of the doctor's shirt or the kind of glasses he or she wore. They always vividly remember the date and can describe the trip to the hospital in explicit detail, but they usually fail to retain any of the important information (Martin et al., 1990).

The value of any diagnostic process can only be as good as the counseling techniques and procedures employed. Of what use is it to have highly accurate tests and highly "efficient" procedures if you cannot communicate them effectively to the clients? Our data indicate that the medical model is not an effective tool, whether it is used by a committee or by individuals. The research cited in Chapter 1 (Lerner, 1988; Martin et al., 1987; Williams & Derbyshire, 1982) has shown how little of the information provided parents retain and how little they trust the audiologist. There are much better ways to conduct a diagnostic examination, which, although they may involve more time in the initial stages, will be much more efficient in the long term. The recommended approach is client centered, as opposed to the institution-centered approach of the medical model.

Client-Centered Diagnosis

For a good diagnostic examination, it is important that the professional understand and have some empathy for the client's history. When clients are first seen in the clinic, they bring with them a long history of their personal struggles with the realization that something is wrong. For example, a scenario for the parents of a child who is congenitally deaf might be something like this: One parent (in this case the mother) becomes aware that something is wrong with the child. The first fear that parents frequently have when they suspect something is wrong is that their child might be mentally retarded. (Retardation is generally what parents fear the most.) When the mother begins to localize the problems to the hearing area, she confides her fears to the father, who responds by denying it, reassuring his wife and himself that nothing is wrong with their baby. At this point, each parent embarks on a surreptitious program of testing the child's hearing without confiding their fears to each other. Now the parents are on an emotional rollercoaster; they are elated when they get a response or a pseudo-response and crushed when the child fails to respond. They often elicit pseudo-responses, for example, by banging pans together behind the child's back (which creates a pressure wave that the child feels or casts a shadow on the wall that is evident within the child's peripheral vision) or by making a sound loud enough that the child responds legitimately even though there is a substantial hearing loss.

The denial mechanism is activated early during this self-diagnosis process so that parents can find many reasons why the child does not respond. (This is equally true for any insidious neurological disease. My wife and I, for example, spent a great deal of time explaining away her vague neurological symptoms; one becomes an expert at finding benign reasons for frighteningly deviant behavior.) This period of uncertainty is very painful as the individuals vacillate between the peaks of relief and the valleys of fear and anxiety. Finally, the denial mechanism, battered by the assault of accumulated data, gives way, and with a great deal of trepidation, the family approaches a professional for a diagnosis of the disorder. At this point, the parents have generally agreed that something is wrong; they sustain themselves with the thought that medical science will be able to cure the disorder. They think that if their child is deaf, an operation or a device will enable the child to hear again. (My wife and I hoped that the neurologist would be able to recommend a drug or a course of action that would cure the disorder or at least prevent further a decline in her functioning. I remember also hoping that he would simply attribute her symptoms to advancing age.) All clients come to the diagnostic situation with the knowledge that there is something wrong but also with some sustaining hope. It is the dashing of this hope that is so painful and that initiates the grief reaction.

Clients are always anxious when they arrive at the clinic. They do not know what to expect; they are hoping that they are wrong. They have composed a story detailing their experiences and they need to be allowed a chance to tell it to someone who will listen to them. It is essential that they be given a chance to tell their story. A question such as, "Can you tell me what brought you here?" will generally elicit the story.

Client-centered counseling in the diagnostic process begins at the moment of initial contact with the family and is continuous throughout the relationship. What needs to be established at the outset is the parents' major concern and their expectations of the professional. Typically, parents express some concern about the child's hearing or speech. At this point, I don't try to get a case history from the parents; I simply let them tell me anything they think is important. I will get to the more specific details later in the process.

After the parents have shared their concerns and told their story, we all must have a clear idea of what we are trying to accomplish on that day. This is known as contracting. The usual "contract" we arrive at is to find out the child's hearing status. Any other contract has to be carefully negotiated. I then enlist the parents as coworkers, saying something such as, "I may be an expert on the testing of hearing, but you are certainly an expert on this child; I need your help."

This remark about needing help is not a ploy to get parents involved but is very much the truth. Parents have a great deal of information about the child that can be used in the diagnostic process. Parents can come to the testing with most of the information in hand. Dale (1991) found that parents' self-reports of the vocabulary and syntax of their 2-year-old children correlated .79 with the results of standardized tests administered to the children. He strongly recommended that parents' self-reports be used in speech and language evaluations because he found them to be

1. more representative of infant and toddler language than laboratory samples;

2. cost-effective for a rapid general evaluation of child language;

3. helpful in selecting assessment procedures for more in-depth analyses, if they are used before the child is seen; and

4. useful for monitoring changes that may result from intervention.

But above all, the self-report, which enlists the parents as codiagnosticians, begins the process of empowering them. When I conduct the audiological examination, I also bring in any other family members who have accompanied the parents, including grandparents and siblings. If it gets too chaotic, I may ask the other family members to leave, but often they are very helpful, especially if there is an older sibling I can use as a model to condition the child being diagnosed. I start testing the child, usually giving one parent the audiogram to fill out. In this way, the information they need is being incorporated into what they are doing and seeing. The audiogram becomes much more meaningful to them because they are using it. When I test an adult, I usually have a family member in the test module with me who fills in the audiogram and scores the speech discrimination tests. I strongly suggest that the adult with a hearing impairment be accompanied by a family member when making an appointment for the examination.

When a sound comes on, I describe how loud it is in terms of decibels and in terms of environmental stimuli (e.g., "This sound is about as loud as people talk"). Then I ask the parents whether they thought their child heard the sound. Depending on the age of the child, we might use visual reinforcement audiometry, where a light is paired with a sound, or play audiometry, where the child is conditioned to respond to a particular sound, for example, by placing a block in a toy mailbox. If the parents and I disagree, I present the sound again until we have some agreement. At the end of the testing, I ask the parents what they think about their child's hearing, and we decide whether the child has a hearing loss. If we cannot agree, we continue testing, or if the child is not cooperative, we decide on a Scotch verdict of "not proven" and schedule another appointment. I never overrule the parents' opinion. Although I might hold to my opinion that the child does have a hearing loss, I never impose it on the parents; they would lose too much power if I did this and would not be fully invested in the child's habilitation program.

Years later, parents have recounted to me the feelings they had experienced during this kind of testing process. They frequently reported how painful it was to sit in the room and hear those loud sounds while their child showed no response. This procedure diminishes the denial mechanism because the parents actually witness the hearing impairment. There is no way out for them because the testing procedure is modified according to their perceptions, and they are the ones who actually do the diagnosis.

Clinical procedures that separate the families from the testing process frequently increase denial because the parents can fantasize about the testing (i.e., maybe the machine was broken or tracings were switched or . . .). Although procedures that separate the parents might be more clinically accurate in detecting and determining the hearing loss because there are no distractions for the audiologist, they are worthless if the parents cannot or will not accept the results. Parents have a need to "view the body." There is tremendous folk wisdom in the traditional funeral ritual when people go to the funeral parlor and view a body in the open casket, accompany the hearse to the cemetery, and watch the casket be lowered into the open grave. This might seem cruel, but it is psychologically sound because it diminishes the denial reaction and allows the grief process to begin. The needed restructuring of one's life because of the loss can then begin. Among the people in our society who are more psychologically disabled are the members of the families of Vietnam War veterans who are still missing in action. These individuals cannot commit fully to a new life because they have not participated in a funeral. There is always a part of them that expects their loved ones to return, and they can imagine all sorts of scenarios in which the loved ones might still be alive. Denial in this case forestalls grief and delays or diminishes the necessary restructuring.

Active parental involvement in the diagnostic process not only diminishes the denial mechanism, it also strengthens the bond between the audiologist and the parents. Parents have reported to me how glad they were that I was there helping them through the painful process. I was seen as an ally rather than as an adversary. No matter how nicely they do it, audiologists who deliver to parents in the waiting room the word that their child is deaf are often received with hostility. People are prone to killing the messenger when they don't like the message.

Another benefit of having the parents as collaborators in the diagnostic process is that they are also being educated about their child's hearing status. The information is gradually delivered to them, and because they are participating, it is retained much more readily than when a professional delivers a "taped" speech at the end of the testing to parents who have been sitting in the waiting room. Participating parents not only understand audiograms better, they also obtain an idea of what this child can and cannot hear in the home environment—information that becomes very useful for them in the habilitation process. Participating in this way is especially helpful for the families of adults because it lets them see the extent of the disability and enables them to effectively collaborate in the habilitation process. I think no adult should be seen without a participating family member. If we are to provide truly family-centered assistance, it must begin at the diagnostic intake.

If, after completing the testing, we decide that the child does have a hearing impairment, I do not supply gratuitous information. Although I know that parents "need" a lot more information to effectively manage their child's habilitation than I give on that first session, I also know that at this point I can't overwhelm them with content. I ask the parents, "What do you need to know now?" and I allow them to guide their own learning experience. I usually get a few desultory questions, which I answer simply because I know that the parents are in a state of shock. This is true even when parents come in telling you that they think their child is deaf. Parents have told me that after the definitive diagnosis, which confirmed their worst fears, all they wanted to do was go someplace and cry.

Sometimes the parents actually respond to the diagnosis with relief, first, because it is deafness and not retardation, of which they were afraid, and second, because somebody finally believed them and gave a name to their child's strange behaviors. People sometimes think that having put a name to the problem means there is a way of controlling it. When they realize that there is no cure and that their child will be deaf for the rest of his or her life, the active grieving begins.

Over the years, I have found that one cannot go any faster with a child than the parents are willing or able to go. Audiologists limit truly effective case management when they become overwhelmed by their own anxiety to get the habilitation process moving. They often try to bypass the parental grief reaction by taking active management of the case, leading invariably to passive, dependent parents and to ineffective long-term management of the child. I feel very strongly that if we pay careful attention to the parents during the diagnostic process by taking time for them and giving them space to grieve, then the child will do well in the long term. This may require the audiologist to let time elapse between the diagnosis and the initiation of habilitation procedures. It is difficult for most audiologists, however, to see a child needing services and not getting them immediately.

Recently I came across a poem written by a professional and a parent that captures the essence of the interpersonal, affective dimension of the diagnostic process:

Advice to Professionals Who Must Conference Cases

Before the case conference,
I would look at my almost 5-year-old son
And see a golden-haired boy
Who giggled at his new baby sister's attempt to clap her hands,
Who charmed adults by his spontaneous hugs and hello's,
Who captured his parents with his rapture with music and his care for white-
haired people who walked a walk a bit slower than younger folks,
Who often became a legend in places visited because of his exquisite ability
to befriend a few special souls,
Who often wanted to play "peace marches,"
And who, at the age of 4,
went to the Detroit Public Library
requesting a book on Martin Luther King.

After the case conference,
I looked at my almost 5-year-old son.
He seemed to have lost his golden hair.
I saw only words plastered on his face.
Words that drowned us in fear and revolting nausea.

Words like:
Primary expressive speech and language disorder
severe visual–motor delay
sensory integration dysfunction
fine- and gross-motor delay
developmental dyspraxia and
RITALIN now.

I want my son back. That's all
I want him back now. Then I'll get on with my life.
If you could feel the depth of this wrenching pain.
If you could see the depth of our sadness
then you would be moved to return
our almost 5-year-old son
who sparkles in the sunlight despite
his faulty neurons.

Please give me back my son
undamaged and
untouched by your labels, test results,
descriptions and categories

If you can't
If you truly cannot give us back our son

Then
just be with us quietly,
gently,
and compassionately as we feel.

Just sit patiently
and attentively as
we grieve and feel powerless.

Sit with us and create a stillness known only in small, empty
chapels at sundown.
Be there
With us as our witness and as our friend.

Please do not give us
advice,
suggestions,
comparisons or
another appointment. (That's for later.)

We want only
a quiet shoulder
upon which to rest our too-heavy heads.

If you can't give us back our sweet dream
then
comfort us through this nightmare.

Hold us.
Rock us
until morning light creeps in.

Then we will rise
and begin the work of a new day.

—Janice Fialka, parent, MSW, ACSW
(Copyright 1994 by the author. Reprinted with permission.)

The second question I ask parents when we emerge from the test booth is "Can you share with me how you are feeling?" This is an invitation to talk about affect. I sometimes give parents a bit of help by saying, "Some parents at this time feel like they have been hit by a truck," or "Some parents feel like they are walking through someone else's nightmare." Occasionally, parents begin to cry and I stay with them. My own experience has led me to believe that the parents who cry most at the initial diagnostic session do better than those parents who seem to accept the diagnosis stoically. The criers are usually not very adept at using denial, and they are realizing the extent of the disability rather quickly. After the initial falling apart, they usually recover quite well and get readily to work. The stoics very often are buttressed by denial and sometimes never make it out of denial to work effectively with their child.

A frequent mistake audiologists make with parents of a child who has a relatively mild hearing loss is to try to cheer up the parents by saying it could be much worse. First, it is always a mistake to try to cheer up people in pain because it invalidates their feelings. The message received is that they have no right to feel badly. Second, the degree of disability is always in the eyes of the beholder. To these parents, the disorder is very severe, and their feeling needs to be respected and not minimized. At this point, the parents need someone to listen to them nonjudgmentally and someone who is not trying to focus their attention on content that they cannot absorb.

I leave parents of newly diagnosed children with the name and phone number of parents of an older child with a hearing impairment (they seldom call at first, as they are still in denial), and I set up an appointment to see them within a week. I may reframe the situation for parents by saying that they are now guaranteed to have an interesting life—not the one they thought they were going to have, but an interesting one nonetheless. In subsequent appointments I supply more information as the parents ask for it and seem ready to receive it. I start each session with that same question: "What do you need to know now?" I have found that the parents eventually ask all of the important questions. They might not be in the same order that would occur if I were in complete control of the content, but the important issues are covered. Parents ask each question when they are ready for the answer. Although it may take a bit longer to get the hearing aid on the child or to have the child enrolled in an educational program than if I had taken initial control, these things will happen nonetheless. It is important that these are accomplished with the support of parents who have taken responsibility and have actively participated in the educational decisions regarding their child and are therefore more likely to follow through on good educational management practices.

Speech–language pathologists can conduct diagnostic evaluations of children in the same way. For example, in a speech or language evaluation, parents can be enlisted as codiagnosticians and experts on their child's behavior, and they can score the test results or elicit responses from the child. This empowers as well as educates the parents. For adult patients, it is necessary to empower the spouse (or significant other) as well as the client. I always bring spouses into the audiometric test booth and sometimes have them give the hearing test or mark the audiogram. Clients always select their own hearing aids and guide all aspects of their testing. Rollins (1988) conducted examinations of patients with aphasia using the spouse as the active tester and the speech–language pathologist as the "coach." Counseling became much easier when the family participated actively in obtaining the diagnostic information.

One question that emerges very quickly once the diagnosis is agreed upon is the cause of the disorder. Handling this question is a very delicate counseling issue. One must determine responsibility without affixing blame. Parents who are obsessed with finding the cause are usually obsessed with guilt. They are looking to find a "cause" that is not their guilty secret. Each parent may be looking to blame the spouse or anyone else. It is very tricky handling this situation, and the careful clinician must steer a course between the "Scylla" of blame and the "Charybdis" of uncertainty. In order to have a successful outcome, parents must give up the past and the search for the cause and deal constructively with their "now." It is often fruitful to begin to explore the guilt issue at this time, although it may be hard to elicit. Often the unasked question is the one we need to answer. "What caused my baby's deafness?" is really "What did I do to cause my baby to be deaf?" Unless we address the unasked question that reflects the parent's feeling of guilt, he or she will be stuck searching for the cause. This search is usually fruitless and a waste of energy that can be better spent in service of the child.

True are some parents who don't seem to react at all to the diagnosis of a hearing loss in their child. In families in which a great many negative things have happened, the deafness is just one more thing. In the Emerson College nursery, we recently had a child of a family in which the husband/father had left. The mother and her three children were now homeless and penniless. This mother had minimal physical and emotional energy to devote to dealing with her daughter's deafness. When told of the hearing loss, she responded with resignation.

People show their feelings in different ways. Some families and some cultures believe that it is inappropriate to display feelings publicly. These families seem to not react to the diagnosis, although they may be deeply pained. Clinicians must not project their feelings onto parents and expect all families to respond in the way they would if they had just found out that their child had a disability. It is very easy to become judgmental; this must be avoided at all costs.

I see the diagnostic occasion as the first step on the long journey that our clients have before them. If we do our job well, we can make that a giant step and help the clients avoid many pitfalls that await them. We can also make it much easier for the professionals who are further down the clients' habilitation road.

Summary

The following is a list of the seven steps needed for a healthy, client-centered diagnostic process.

1. Allow the client and family to tell their story. Use of an open-ended question such as "What brought you here?" is usually very helpful.

2. Enlist the family as collaborators. Empower them with a statement, for example, "You are the expert on this child, and I'll be the expert on the testing."

3. Actively involve the family and client in the testing procedure. The client should have choices where possible, and the family can be active in eliciting or scoring responses.

4. Have the client and family participate fully in the final diagnosis. In an ideal situation, they will make the diagnosis.

5. Empower them by asking, "What do you need to know now?" Let them guide you as to how much information you should give.

6. Listen and respond to the affect. Give clients a chance to talk about how they feel in an unhurried, caring atmosphere. If there is a time limit, then tell the family this at the outset, for example, "I have 15 minutes before my next appointment; how can I be helpful to you?"

7. Set up another appointment. Do not try to cover everything in one appointment. If this is not possible, help them locate additional support in the form of peer counseling.

Institution-Initiated Diagnosis

As mentioned in the introduction, because of the advent of universal hearing screening of newborns, we are moving from a parent-initiated model of diagnosis to an institution-initiated model. Instead of a parent gradually becoming aware of their child's disability and seeking an explanation, the professional now has the obligation to inform a totally unaware parent of the deficit. The timing of newborn screening programs could not be worse. There is never a good time to tell parents of their child's possible disability, but I could not think of a worse time than 1 or 2 days postpartum. At that point, parents have been through the ordeal of birth, hormones are running amok, and they need time to physically and emotionally recover so as to bond with their baby. They are certainly not ready to receive bad news. Unfortunately, many screening programs require that parents be told of their child's problem before leaving the hospital. I think this is a big mistake. I think parents will be more receptive to the diagnosis if they are given a respite and informed at a later time, preferably by a professional who already has a relationship with them—such as the family pediatrician—or a professional who can give them information—such as the audiologist. An unintended consequence of newborn screening has been to distance the audiologist from the immediate diagnosis.

In data I and my associate Kurtzer-White have been gathering from parents of children with hearing impairments who have failed the screening, we found that not one parent was told of the failure by an audiologist. Instead, they were informed by hospital personnel, none of whom could supply the parents with any information other than the test results. Instead of going home to enjoy their babies, these parents went home to worry and to test their infant's hearing. In many cases, it was several months before they could get an appointment to confirm the loss. In the words of one mother, "It was just Hell." Horror stories abound: parents finding out by seeing a note on their child's bassinet or being told as they are leaving the hospital by a nurse that "Your baby failed the screening test but don't worry about it." "And of course," said the mother, "That is all I worried about." In a published study, Luterman and Kurtzer-White (1999) found that what parents of children who are deaf want the most at the time of diagnosis is to meet other parents get help with their feelings, and be given unbiased information. Unfortunately, none of the parents in our sample whose child had failed the screening received any of the things they needed; instead, they were left with a quasi-diagnosis and no place to go.

This is not necessarily a failure of screening as it is a failure to establish a good and humane management component. I think newborn screening can be an integral part of a comprehensive habilitation program if we devise suitable management procedures that are in accord with good counseling principles. The following are my suggestions:

The notification of screening failure should be taken out of the hospital, where the audiologist has no control of the process. Instead, the pediatrician should be informed, and he or she can closely question the parents on their first visit. (This requires educating pediatricians about the identification of hearing loss. We can do this with the money we save on eliminating many of the false positives by deferring the second test.) By doing this, we give the parents some time to recover from the birth process and also time to bond with their baby. If there is some doubt in the pediatrician's mind or the parents' minds after they have been questioned, the pediatrican should refer the family for further testing.

Pediatricians need to be told not to use the word "failure" in telling the parent. Instead, they should tell parents that this is a two-part test, and the second part needs to be completed. Using this procedure ensures that the parents are alerted by a professional who has some relationship with them within their "medical home." I think this a more humane way of managing screening than current procedures seem to be. I suspect we will also get a higher compliance rate than we currently have.

Appointments to the audiologist must be fast-tracked so that a minimum amount of time occurs between when the pediatrician informs the parents and the audiological appointment. Audiologists can then proceed with good diagnostic practice as outlined previously in this chapter. At all times, audiologists must try to employ clinical procedures that involve the parents and objectify the hearing loss, which is not easy to do with an infant but is well worth the effort. Once the diagnosis is confirmed, good counseling procedures based on a listening and valuing model should be employed.

CHAPTER

Techniques of Counseling

I approached writing this chapter with some trepidation. If students concentrate solely on their counseling technique, their effectiveness can be severely limited. Good counseling technique flows from personality—it is seamless. Technique should not be apparent to the person being counseled or to an observer. If people know they are being counseled, you are probably doing it wrong. This is not to say that there is no technique or that there is no discipline to be learned by the student. As the counselor gains more experience and becomes more secure, technique is incorporated into personality; the skill then becomes unconscious. I find that I frequently have to invent a reason why I did something when a student observer questions me in postevaluation sessions. Counseling is something I just "do." If I am conscious of technique, I become mechanical, and the technique fails because it interferes with the authenticity of the relationship.

Counseling is not a mantle that the professional puts on when a client is present and then discards the rest of the time. It is an attitude, something that is lived. I do not see how one can be a caring, responsive person only within the context of a client–professional relationship and not in other aspects of one's life. Counseling, as I view it, is an integrated approach to all interpersonal relationships: One "counsels" everybody who approaches in a caring and responsive manner. The techniques employed by a counselor will flow from personality and personal congruence as well as from a counseling philosophy that has been incorporated into the way in which the counselor approaches clients. Each counselor develops a personal-paradigms framework of thought: a personal strategy for understanding and explaining certain aspects of reality that could be considered a filter built from an individual's life experiences, prejudices, and constructs. A paradigm is the central organizer of how each person views reality. Events are filtered through our personal paradigms and interpreted by us. In counseling, our paradigms are influenced very heavily by our philosophical notions of how people learn.

In Chapter 2, I discussed four somewhat different ways of viewing the client. The behaviorist sees the client as a mass of conditioned responses. The humanist sees an organism that is seeking to grow. The existentialist sees someone struggling with the great issues of existence (death, freedom, loneliness, and meaninglessness). The cognitivist sees someone who has made unfounded intellectual assumptions about the world that need to be examined.

Technique should not be bound to a particular philosophy. Although I like to think of myself as a humanist, I use some techniques that fit well within behavioral or rational–emotive therapy. I think a professional should not make therapeutic choices because of identification with a particular therapy but because the evidence based on clinical experience has tended to indicate that this is the way to be most helpful to the client. Arbuckle (1970) wrote the following passage about this subject:

> In the long run, it would seem that the effective counselor is one who has worked out for himself, through the experience of experimentation, the means by which he can most effectively use himself in the human interaction known as counseling. His orientation has been eclectic, rather than parochial and while his own life is in a constant state of movement and change, he has learned that there are certain modes of operation, which are most effective for him, thus there is a degree of consistency in his operation as a counselor. While he is open to consider any means that will work with the client, he is aware that his own limitations are such that he cannot be all things for all people. He is acceptant of the thought that there is no model, no method, no technique, which will be consistently successful for him with any other human individual who may come to him as a client. (p. 291)

Counselor Control Via Response

In a counseling relationship, I wait to hear what issues are on the client's mind before I make a clinical judgment concerning how best to proceed. There are no stupid questions, only ill-judged responses. The nondirective or person-centered approach affords a great deal of counselor control. The way the counselor elects to respond will to a large extent determine the future course of the counselor–client interaction. The timing of a response is critical: Sometimes a client can make good use of content; at other times, the content is very inappropriate. The counselor needs to select the response that will be most facilitative within the context of client interaction. It is only through careful listening that the counselor can do this. If the counselor listens carefully, the client will tell him or her what is needed.

For example, a father of a child who is deaf might say, "There are no adequate services for deaf children in this state." I might respond to this statement in one of the following ways:

- telling him about the services that are available and offering him a directory of services (content response);
- asking him how he came to have that opinion (counterquestion);
- saying, "That must frighten you when you think about the lack of available services for your child" (affect response);
- telling him he is correct, and then commenting on what a wonderful opportunity this presents for him to get involved in establishing suitable programs (reframing);
- telling him about my experience trying to find services for my child (sharing self); or
- responding with a clinical "uh huh" (affirmation).

None of these responses is necessarily the best one. (I have chosen six possible responses that seem to be the most clinically facilitative.) Each response is appropriate within the context of the relationship. Each response will move the relationship into a different dimension, and the appropriateness is determined by a clinical judgment of the therapeutic context. The timing of the response is critical, as are many nonverbal features—tone of voice, facial expression, and body language. I want to look at each response in a bit more detail.

Content Response

The content response—the one most commonly used by professionals—generally keeps the relationship at an expected and rather predictable level. In the initial stages of a relationship, the professional provides content to establish credibility; in the latter stages, content is necessary for the making of appropriate decisions. Generally, content-based relationships are short term and fall under the medical model of service delivery. When the professional has a limited amount of time, content predominates and tends to keep waiting rooms clear. It also keeps the client in a cognitive realm and away from feelings. A professional does have the responsibility to keep current regarding information in his or her area and to separate fact from opinion—not an easy task. Content has immense value when it is used appropriately.

Counterquestion

I have found that people seldom want advice. They usually seek confirmation of a position or a decision that they have already made. Instead of revealing that decision, they often ask a question in hopes that their decision will be confirmed by me. Giving advice rarely works: A wise man doesn't need it, and a fool won't take it. I have a sign over my desk that says, "Give me a fish and I eat for a day. Teach me to fish and I eat for the rest of my life." Advice giving is fish giving. People don't learn from it. If it works, they are back for more, and if it fails, they curse the giver of the advice, but in either case they have not learned. Often the most productive and facilitative response one can give to a confirmation question is the counterquestion.

The counterquestion forces the person to reveal his or her position. If one treats a confirmation question as a content question, then one is very likely to put one's foot in one's mouth. For example, a Spanish-speaking mother of a boy who had just been diagnosed as deaf asked me whether she would have to speak English to him at home if she enrolled her child in the Emerson College nursery. I resisted the temptation to tell her that it would be less confusing for her child if she did (she could figure that out for herself) and instead responded by asking her what she wanted to do. The woman responded that if we made her speak English at home, she would not enroll in the nursery. I told her our policy was to speak English in the nursery and that she could decide what she wanted to do at home. The mother accepted that, and a month later, when she was ready, she announced to the parent support group that she was going to speak English at home. (At the time of admission to the program, she was not ready to give up her child as both a deaf child and a non–Spanish-speaking child. Parents will always find the "right" answer if we give them time and space to do it.)

It was a relief to me to realize that I did not have to answer questions. (I think this was a holdover from my school days, when I was rewarded by answering my teacher's questions and thus could prove how smart I was.) The counterquestion is a very valuable teaching strategy. It forces the learner back onto his or her own resources. The counterquestion response to the client's lament, "You don't answer my questions," is "Why should I answer your questions?"

Confirmation questions also are used to forestall rejection. A question is a low-risk contribution to an interaction: The questioner does not have to reveal himself or herself; instead, he or she is asking the other person to make a revelation. For example, when I am asked if I am busy tonight, I usually respond by asking if the questioner had something in mind for me to do. Embedded in almost all questions is a statement, and I need to be sensitive enough to respond to the statement or at least to elicit it.

For me, the best indicator of the trust level in a professional–client relationship is the number of question–answer interactions. In initial stages of a relationship, where trust is not high, there are usually a great many questions. As the relationship develops and grows, the client becomes more willing to offer statements and observations. The professional can facilitate this therapeutic movement by not always answering questions and supplying content. The counterquestion can be a powerful tool for moving the relationship beyond the initial stages.

Affect Response

On the surface, the affect response appears risky, but actually it is responding to what Carl Rogers in a filmed lecture called "the faint knocking." By listening very carefully and trying to see the world as the client sees it and reflecting the feelings back, the counselor can help to open up the relationship—sometimes very dramatically. The appropriate affect response greatly increases the intimacy level in a relationship. I have found that even an inaccurate response is not harmful; it generally forces people to clarify further their feelings, and in the process of clarification, we both can generally understand the feelings better.

The affect response is very potent in building a counseling relationship. Caring is conveyed by our willingness to listen and be responsive to what the person says and also to what the person cannot quite bring himself or herself to say. Rogers (1951) called this *empathetic listening*, which at first glance would appear to be a readily teachable technique. Unfortunately, empathetic listening is often abused and can come across as parroting or mechanical in the hands of someone who has learned the form but not the substance of the humanistic approach. In an article written for physicians, Sabbeth and Leventhal (1988) talked about the "trial balloons" that patients and families send up when they interact with their doctor, asserting that it is the physician's responsibility to respond to the feelings imbedded in those balloons. I remember one family with whom I worked in which the husband had had a severe stroke. Almost as an aside, the wife said, "I can't seem to leave the house anymore without going back to check whether I have locked the door and shut off the stove. Sometimes

I go back two or three times." My response to her was, "It seems like you don't trust yourself." This led to a very fruitful discussion of her anxiety and feelings of inadequacy regarding her ability to cope with her husband's disabilities.

Because the affect response requires considerable follow up, it should rarely be given if the professional has only a limited amount of time. I find that responding at the affect level is usually more appropriate in the initial stages of contact and diagnosis. It allows for a ventilation of emotions and for the alleviation of some of the secondary feelings that accompany the strong affect surrounding a catastrophic illness. For example, the wife who feels very angry at her husband for having a stroke can be given the opportunity to talk about her feelings of anger without feeling guilty. In later stages, when affect is not predominant, I generally give more content responses or reframe experiences into something more positive.

Reframing

The timing of reframing has to be precise, and it cannot be used too frequently, or the professional will be accused of being a "Pollyanna." It is immensely effective in mobilizing the person to look at the positive side of a situation. Good reframing always gives the person a jolt. It should cause him or her to stop short and examine the assumptions underlying his or her statement. As professionals, we are so focused on the problem that we seldom see the challenge. Reframing encourages responsibility assumption. The parent who complains about the "dumb questions" he or she gets from strangers who see the child's hearing aids can be brought up short by the response, "What a marvelous opportunity to educate someone about deafness."

Professionals can also benefit from the reframing response by looking for the positive when analyzing their client relationships. For example, behavior can be interpreted as stubborn or as determined. If the clinician is always looking at the client's stubborn side, he or she will have a negative view of the client.

I think that we seldom consider or call attention to a client's strengths because we are often looking at the deficits. When I supervise student clinicians, it helps to ask them, "What does this child have going for him?" and "How can we capitalize on those strengths?" When we focus on the client's strengths, the problem begins to disappear far faster than when we emphasize the deficits. It might seem that there are limits to situations that can be reframed, but this may not be so. I remember watching a video of Kubler-Ross counseling a woman in the terminal stages of amyotrophic lateral sclerosis. She was totally paralyzed and being cared for by her two daughters. Through one of her daughters, who bent close to her barely moving lips, she asked Kubler-Ross,

"What good am I?" and Kubler-Ross's response, without batting an eye, was, "You are giving your daughters a chance to pay you back for all the care you gave them," which seemed to satisfy the woman.

I have several favorite reframings to the question, "Why me?" I might respond, "Why not you?" To families with children who have just been diagnosed as having a disability, I might say, "This child has guaranteed you an interesting life." I try to reframe all "mistakes" into "nuggets of gold" whereby the person learned something valuable. I might comment to a client that his disability is a powerful teacher for him (and can be for others as well). I have personally found this idea of teacher in disability very potent. It also works with interpersonal and clinical relationships. I can reframe difficult clients into potent teachers for me, and I can do the same with previously obnoxious colleagues and acquaintances. If I approach them as people who have something to give me so that I grow, the quality of the interaction changes markedly. For the astute business person, the complaining customer is his or her best friend because that customer is helping improve the product. With such an attitude, you can change the world.

Reframing as a technique and as a life tool is very powerful. For all of the possible responses, but especially reframing, the timing is critical. It is very easy to lose people by reframing too early in the grief process; an ill-timed or ill-delivered response can be very offensive. On the other hand, the ultimate goal of counseling is to help the clients reframe their life situations into something positive. When they do this themselves, the counselor's job is finished because there is no longer any problem.

Sharing Self

The image of the professional is often of someone who is always in total control; someone who knows the answers and therefore someone whom the client admires. In practice, we know this is not true, that there are times when we the professionals are out of control in both our personal and professional lives. Standard clinical practice says we should hide this from our clients. I have found, however, that it is sometimes very helpful and facilitative to share my own doubts and uncertainties with clients. If we always seem in control, clients tend to feel inadequate. A father of a child with Down's syndrome said, "I like to see the teacher have a hard time with my son. It validates my experience too." When he comes over to to fix something that my ineptitude has caused, I tell my son to struggle a bit before he fixes it so I won't feel so badly. Unfortunately, he doesn't always do this, and my feeling of inadequacy is reinforced. Sometimes the most helpful thing we can say to a parent might be, "I haven't the foggiest idea what to do right now with your child. Do you have any ideas?" This empowers the parent and humanizes us at the same time.

Sharing self also means being willing to tell clients that we are angry with them. This is an opportunity to work out issues in the relationship. Change comes about because of conflict resolution. If we do not allow conflict to emerge by sharing feelings, we will be stuck in relationships that are ultimately unsatisfying. Few professionals ever let themselves be angry with clients directly. More often, they vent on colleagues or repress the anger, which usually subverts the therapy. Similarly, we don't always share our positive feelings with clients. Sharing the self reveals our authenticity as fellow human beings in a meaningful relationship with our clients.

It is valuable to the clients to realize that the professional is also a person who has concerns, fears, and a life outside of the clinic. This revelation helps the client assume responsibility and prevents the professional from being elevated to miracle worker status. The timing of this response is especially critical. If it is done too early, the professional will lose credibility at a time when credibility establishment is critical to the relationship. The sharing responses should usually emerge later in the relationship and with clients who have a relatively high degree of self-esteem.

Affirmation

I am reminded of a certain cartoon featuring a psychoanalyst: A patient is on the couch talking, and the psychiatrist is asleep; presumably, progress is being made. Very often the client just needs a sounding board; he or she needs permission to talk and to express feelings without judgment. The "uh huh" response, accompanied by appropriate nonverbal behavior, can be very helpful in unleashing the client's feelings. This is not just being silent, it involves the counselor who must be listening carefully so that he or she is fully "present" for the client and a witness to the client's struggle. The "uh huh" is also an affirmation that the counselor has heard the client and an invitation for the client to continue. In my office I have a poster given to me by a group of students that says, "It often shows a fine command of language to say nothing." Sometimes the most facilitative remarks are the ones that you do not deliver.

Choosing a Response

The clinician has a wide array of potential responses; which one is selected can determine the direction of the client relationship. There are no "right" responses, only different ones. If the response you give moves the relationship in a fruitful direction, it is appropriate. It is also quite possible to recover from taking the wrong road. I have found that if something is important, it keeps coming up. A feeling is seldom lost—It gets reworked and emerges again.

The following selected questions and statements were made by clients and family members. The reader may want to use them to practice the various responses discussed in this chapter. Again, there are no right or wrong answers.

1. If this were your child, what would you do?

2. Are cochlear implants any good?

3. My husband's family is very unemotional.

4. Will I have to be present when you test my husband?

5. Is it true that graduates of schools for the deaf are only able to read on a third-grade level?

6. What causes stuttering in a child?

7. Is the school for children with developmental delays a good school?

8. Do we have to drill on the [s] sound any more?

9. My wife can't stand the sound of the artificial larynx.

10. I am so afraid of making a bad decision for this child.

11. You don't answer any of my questions.

12. I often think about my husband dying.

CASE STUDIES: HYPOTHETICAL FAMILIES

The hypothetical families presented here are fictionalized case studies designed to illuminate particular problems. I have used them in classes I teach to speech–language pathology majors, in inservice workshops, and less frequently in parent groups. I found them very useful for me in my early work with groups when I needed the comfort of more structure and direction in my role as the leader. I seldom use them now because I prefer a much less-structured experience.

The first 10 of the following case studies have been adapted from a *Volta Review* article (Luterman, 1969). The case studies can be rewritten (I have done this with several) to reflect any disability. The original cases all involved deafness, but the problems illuminated by the case studies are universal. Interested readers may use the cases as is or may alter them to suit the needs of a particular group.

1. Mrs. A. is very confused. She has taken her $2\frac{1}{2}$-year-old son, who is neither talking nor seeming to respond to sound, to several physicians. Her pediatrician has told her that he thought her child was deaf but that nothing could be done until he was 4 years old. One physician has told her that he thinks the child is mentally retarded. Her husband and her in-laws, on the other hand, feel that there is nothing wrong with the child and that he will "outgrow it." They tell her about an uncle who did not begin talking until he was 4 years of age and who is now perfectly normal. What should Mrs. A. do?

2. Mrs. B. sometimes says to herself, "Why did this happen to me?" She has said, "I know I shouldn't feel this way, but I really resent having a deaf child. He takes so much of my energy and time. He is so difficult for me to control; I worry about him so much. Every now and then, I find myself wishing for a moment that I had never had him, and then I feel guilty about feeling that way. I also hate to go out with him because of his screaming and because of the stares of passersby when they see his hearing aid. I just can't stand the questions of strangers and their well-meaning advice any longer." What can be done about Mrs. B.'s feelings?

3. Mrs. C. feels that her deaf child was given to her because of her past "sins." She has devoted herself to taking care of her child; she no longer goes out socially and has dropped most of her friends. She spends a good part of the day working with the deaf child and taking him to his therapy lessons; she spends evenings reading and talking about deafness. She does not trust any babysitters. Mr. C. has begun to complain about feeling neglected, and he says he is concerned about the two older children, who have not received much attention from their mother. What are your feelings about the C. family?

4. Dr. D. is a physician whose father and grandfather were also doctors. He has always wanted to have a son who would be a physician too. Since he has learned that his only child is deaf and therefore will never be able to be a physician, Dr. D. has not devoted much attention to the boy. He has said, "I had so many plans for him. Every time I see the hearing aid, it reminds me that he won't be what I would like him to be, and it's really very hard for me to be with him. I know I shouldn't feel that way and it probably is harmful to him, but having a deaf son is a very big disappointment to me." What can this father do?

5. Mr. and Mrs. E. have three children. Their youngest is a 2-year-old deaf child; the other two are 6 and 10 years of age. The E.'s have been very busy taking the 2-year-old to various clinics for evaluations, and they have begun a twice-weekly therapy program and lessons at home. The middle child has responded to his younger brother's problem very well and, in fact, seems more understanding of it than the old-

est boy. The oldest child has reacted with a great deal of jealousy. He is extremely difficult to manage; he throws violent tantrums and often simply withdraws for fairly long periods of time. Mr. E. has reacted to that behavior with stiff disciplinary measures. Mrs. E.'s reactions have varied from anger to pleading and bribing. At the same time, she recognizes that neither she nor her husband is handling the 10-year-old effectively. What might they do?

6. Mr. and Mrs. F. have a 2-year-old son who is deaf. Mrs. F.'s parents live very near them, and Mrs. Z. has not accepted the fact that her grandson is deaf and will "never" be able to hear. She keeps sending her daughter articles from newspapers and magazines about operations and cures for deafness. She is constantly urging her daughter to take him to one more doctor. Mrs. F. says, "It is hard enough for us to accept our child's deafness, but it is especially difficult when we keep having to explain it over and over again to other people who don't really listen to us." Mr. F.'s parents, on the other hand, live farther away and see their grandchild rather infrequently. When they do see their grandson, they feel he should not be punished— "After all, he is deaf." They become upset if either Mr. or Mrs. F. disciplines the deaf child in their presence. How could that family be helped to reduce some of these conflicts?

7. Timothy G. is a $3\frac{1}{2}$-year-old child who is deaf with no siblings. He is not permitted outside the house unless accompanied by one of his parents, despite the fact that he lives on a quiet suburban street. His mother is very concerned that he might be hit by a child on a bicycle or by a car because he cannot hear. The parents are also afraid that he might fall down and hurt his ear with the hearing aid. Consequently, he seldom leaves his home or plays with children his own age. Should that situation be altered? Why? Why not? If so, what suggestions would you make to the parents?

8. Mr. and Mrs. H. live in a medium-sized town 40 miles from Boston. They have lived in the town all their lives; Mr. H. owns and operates a small business there. The H.'s own their home, and they are both very active in community affairs. They have three children, ages 10, 8, and 5 years, the youngest of whom is deaf and has been accepted in a school for the deaf in a suburb near Boston. Because of the distance involved, the school will accept the child only on a residential basis. Rather than have her daughter board at the school, Mrs. H. wants to move to a community close to the school so that her daughter can attend on a daily basis. Mr. H. is opposed to such a move; he feels that moving to the new community would disrupt the whole family. What should that family do?

9. Mr. and Mrs. I. find themselves at complete odds over the management of their 3-year-old son who is deaf. Mrs. I. is convinced of the worth of the aural–oral approach and is trying to teach her son to lip-read and communicate orally. Mr. I., on the other hand, is convinced that only a very small percentage of persons who are deaf ever attain reasonable oral communication skills. He would prefer that his son learn manual communication so he can at least communicate easily with other per-

sons who are deaf. Mr. I. is around his children very seldom, but whenever he is, he uses manual signs to communicate with his son. What can these parents do?

10. Mr. and Mrs. J. have a 3-year-old child who is deaf. The family lives on an island, and because of the lack of facilities and professional help, Mrs. J. has had the sole responsibility for teaching her daughter. The child is doing well; she lip-reads about 30 words, responds very well to contextual cues, and can use about 15 words expressively. Mrs. J. has placed her child in a nursery school with hearing children, where she also does well; she has just been told that her daughter can begin attending a school for the deaf on the mainland, which means that the child can get home only every 4 to 6 weeks. What should she do?

11. Mr. and Mrs. K. have recently divorced. Mrs. K. has retained custody of their 3-year-old son with autism. The court has given Mr. K. permission to visit the child once a week. Mrs. K. finds that her ex-husband's visits are very unsettling for both her and their son. She feels that her son cannot understand why his father leaves and is not home during the week; the child is very confused by the whole situation. Mr. K. also brings a great many presents when he comes and takes the child to exciting places. Mrs. K. therefore feels that she looks very "bad" to the child, and she is upset at the unfairness of the arrangement. What can this family do to relieve some of the tensions?

12. Mr. and Mrs. L. recently attended an IEP meeting at which the presiding educators unanimously voiced the opinion that their 3-year-old child should go to the local school for the deaf. However, that school only offers a program in total communication. The child has been attending an aural–oral nursery school and has been doing quite well in developing his speech and language skills. The parents want him to continue in the aural mode and would like their child to attend a hearing nursery and receive tutorial help. They believe that the educators are suggesting the school for the deaf because it is expedient and not because it is the best facility for their child. The first IEP meeting ended in a deadlock, and all parties agreed to meet again in 2 weeks. What strategies should the parents employ for the next meeting?

13. Mr. and Mrs. M. have recently found out that their 2-year-old child is deaf. They have one other child, who is older and hears. Mrs. M. has a deaf brother and a deaf uncle; consequently, she feels somehow responsible for the child's deafness. Mr. M. has not been helpful. He also blames Mrs. M. for causing the child's deafness and has left all of the responsibility for the child's education to her. On one level, Mrs. M. deeply resents having that responsibility; on another level, she accepts it as her "punishment." What can Mrs. M. do to alter the unhealthy home situation?

14. The 11-year-old child with cerebral palsy of Mr. and Mrs. N. is deeply resentful of his disability. He is constantly questioning Mr. N. about why he has this problem and refuses to believe that he will not outgrow it. He is currently being mainstreamed and is doing quite well academically; however, he has few friends among the

classmates and he does not want to have anything to do with other people with disabilities. What can Mr. and Mrs. N. do to help their son?

15. Mr. and Mrs. O. are a couple in their 30s who have recently adopted an 18-month-old child, only to discover that the child has multiple disabilities. The adoption is not yet official, and the parents have the option of returning the child to the agency and going on the waiting list for another child. Mrs. O. wants to keep the child because she has grown attached to him and feels that she can be a good parent of a child with disabilities. Mr. O. believes that they should return the child to the agency before they get any more attached. He feels that being a parent is hard enough and that being the parent of a child with disabilities is asking for too much trouble. He is not sure he has the resources to be a good parent to that child, and Mrs. O. feels she cannot raise the child without the full support of her husband. What can that family do?

Locus of Control

Central to all counseling techniques is the concept of locus of control. Rotter (1966), a social psychologist, developed a scale that measures whether an individual has an internal or external locus of control. According to Rotter, people with an internal locus of control tend to feel that they have personal power and can control their own destiny. People with an external locus of control feel that they are controlled by others. "Externals" believe that things just happen to them as the result of luck or fate. "Internals" feel their lives are "them doing them." Locus of control is conceived of as a continuum, with most people located between the extremes of total control (inner locus) and total powerlessness (external locus). Counseling technique, I believe, has to cede control to the client so that ultimately the client feels responsible and empowered to make changes.

Because behaviorists view clients as a mass of conditioned responses controlled by others, behavioral counseling techniques, if used too extensively and inappropriately, tend to encourage clients to have an external locus of control. A careful behavioral counselor teaches the client to identify the reinforcers in the environment and then teaches counterconditioning techniques. Clients in the hands of a competent behavioral therapist can develop an inner locus of control.

Within the sphere of humanistic counseling, control is always vested in the clients. This makes it easier for them to develop an inner locus of control because they have been given control over their learning from the inception of therapy.

The concept of locus of control has received some research attention in communication disorders. Dowaliby, Burke, and McKee (1983) modified the

Rotter (1966) scale for use with individuals with hearing impairment and found that students with hearing impairment who entered college were substantially more external in their locus of control than a control sample of students with normal hearing. White (1982) reported on a series of workshops he conducted with 281 teachers and counselors at six schools for the deaf. The participants were asked to rank 24 social competencies on the basis of what deaf children need to accomplish most. Almost all participants rated "accepting responsibilities for own actions" as the most important issue. Bodner and Johns (1977) used the Rotter scale with 38 students who were deaf and found that they were significantly more external in their locus of control than the control group with normal hearing.

The failure to take responsibility for one's actions in the adult deaf population was recently and vividly brought home to me. I lectured at a conference attended by a large number of adults with hearing impairments, and my speech was interpreted. After the speech, which was an hour long, a man who was sitting in the back of the room complained vigorously that he had missed the entire speech because he could not see the interpreter. The conference organizer, to whom I afterward spoke, felt guilty about the incident until we talked about it, when she realized that the responsibility was not hers. The man could have moved his seat or complained at the onset of the lecture, and the interpreter would have moved. Instead, he made a choice to sit there and then complain about it.

Locus of control has also been studied in people who stutter. Craig, Franklin, and Andrews (1985) used the specially constructed *Locus of Control of Behavior Scale* on 17 persons who stuttered and were in therapy. The researchers found that clients who moved toward internality in locus of control were more likely to maintain improvement over time, whereas relapse was more likely for those who did not internalize. Madison, Budd, and Itzkowitz (1986) found that children who stuttered and who showed greater internality also displayed greater improvement following treatment than did children with a relatively external locus of control.

Locus of control has not been adequately researched in training programs. Only one study stands out. Shirlberg et al. (1977) examined locus of control in college students majoring in communication disorders. They found that the students who had an internal locus of control were rated as the better clinicians. As they so aptly wrote, "Excellent clinicians do in fact view themselves as pilots rather than pawns of their fate" (p. 315).

Populations with disabilities have also been studied in regard to locus of control, and as one might expect, they have generally been found to have an external locus of control. Hallahan, Gasar, Cohen, and Tarver (1978) found that 28 matched teenagers with learning disabilities were significantly more external in their locus-of-control orientation than were control group participants. Land and Vineberg (1965) reported that study participants who were blind were more externally oriented than the nondisabled controls.

The finding of external locus in populations with disabilities is not surprising when one sees how professionals tend to interact with them. It is not uncommon to see professionals who are constantly rescuing clients because they don't want clients to experience additional failure or pain. A clinician who does this promotes an external locus of control that makes populations with disabilities—already dependent for so many things—feel that others are more powerful and more capable than they are.

Encouraging a more internal locus of control in our client populations is as much a matter of attitude as it is of clinical technique. We must convey to clients that they are capable and that they have control over many aspects of their lives. The idea that the client always has control of how he or she will react to the disability is paramount. (Although a person may have no choice about being deaf, he or she always has a choice about what to do about the deafness.) The clinical techniques employed in helping clients generally should be covert and not obvious to them or to observers. Many times we can be most helpful by not doing anything except being there as responsive, caring human beings and allowing the clients to work things out for themselves. Sometimes the very effective clinician creates vacuums that the clients have to fill. Clients are forced to act and to take responsibility for their actions; in doing so, there is growth. Lesson plans, for example, need to be created mutually with the client participating fully in planning the course of therapy. Asking children to choose the toys with which they would like to play, or as mentioned previously, after completing diagnostics, asking the clients what they need to know invests them with some control. In group meetings (discussed in the next chapter), I never call on participants; they are allowed to sit quietly as long as they like. The clinical silence or vacuum becomes a powerful teaching tool that unfortunately is not always appreciated by supervisors.

Language changing is a cognitive technique based on the rational–emotive therapy developed by Ellis (1977), which is more fully described in Chapter 2. Language changing derives from the clinical applications of general semantics. In this technique, the professional pays careful attention to the client's language, which illuminates the underlying and sometimes irrational assumptions the client is making. I have a poster in my office that says, "The shape of my world is the shape of my language." During an interaction I sometimes gently point out to the client the assumption underlying the words he or she is using.

For example, the use of "have to" almost always reflects an external locus of control. When a parent said to me, "I have to try acupuncture," I said, "Don't you mean 'choose to'?" A bit later, I said, "Why do you feel you have to?" This was an invitation for the parent to look at the feeling of being driven and controlled by others. In this particular case, her own guilt was driving her. "But" always reflects an underlying ambivalence. I might respond to a statement such as, "I want to speak in public but I am afraid," with the response, "Can't you be afraid and still speak in public?" This encourages acting in the face of fear; the "but" allows wallowing in ambivalence. I always examine carefully all the "Yes . . . but . . ." statements, which reflect ambivalence. "Should" and "ought" reflect guilt and deficiency. There is always some felt sense of failing when these words are used. Constructs such as, "I should talk to my pediatrician about his incorrect diagnosis of my child's hearing," might receive a response such as, "Do you *want* to talk to your physician?" "Should" and "ought" are also very reflective of an external locus of control, and changing them to "choose to" or "choose not to" encourages a more internal locus and assumption of responsibility for behavior.

We need to help clients recognize the choices they are making. I always examine the clients' language to see where they are evading responsibility. Evasion happens frequently when clients use the pronoun "we" instead of "I," as in "We are unhappy with this class." I might respond, "Do you mean *you* are unhappy?" One indicator of a shift in locus of control is the spontaneous use of the "I" form, which reflects ownership of behavior. When that occurs in clients, I know that we are well on our way to a successful counseling interaction.

When someone says she has been "lucky," I might change the word to "good." If a client says, "I was lucky to have him for a husband," I might respond, "You were good, so therefore he married you." It is very helpful to take credit for the good we do; most "lucky" people take all the responsibility for the bad and very little credit for the good. This is a hard way to live.

I don't allow clients to use collective nouns, such as "men" and "women." When I hear a sentence such as, "All men are lousy," I change it to "The men in my life have been lousy," and then I might gently comment, "It sounds as if you have not been meeting the right men." (I also might comment, "You sound pretty angry.")

Linguistic changes need to be made gently and timing is critical. I seldom make linguistic changes in initial stages of diagnosis or when affect is high because changing languages forces the client into a cognitive stance. The client's trust in the professional also needs to be high, or the linguistic alterations can be seen as interfering and annoying.

Silence

Silence is an important component of any therapeutic relationship. A long, embarrassed silence frequently occurs early in my clinical interactions. Because clients generally expect me, the professional, to direct conversation, when I do not take the lead, a silence ensues. It is vital that I do not break this silence. It tells the client that if he or she wants something to happen in this relationship, he or she has to act. Silence is a primary vehicle for responsibility assumption, and it is vital that I do not take that responsibility from the client. Discomfort with silence initially forces many young clinicians to act; they then become role-bound to make things happen while the client sits back and watches.

In conventional relationships, silences are generally uncomfortable. I can remember the long, painful silences I had as an adolescent on a blind date while I thought frantically of something to say. I suspect the girl was similarly occupied, but I was too concerned with my own discomfort to think of hers. The discomfort generated by clinical silence can be used to motivate action by the client. Because I am fortified by the knowledge of what I am doing and the value of this technique, I can outwait most clients. The general reaction to the silence is anger; if this surfaces, it becomes a useful vehicle for discussing role expectations.

Later in relationships, silences are more reflective and quite comfortable. As intimacy develops, silence becomes a valuable learning time for processing material. Where there is silence, there usually is growth. Cook (1964) analyzed the amount of silences in taped therapy sessions and found that the more successful sessions had more silences than those judged to be less successful. Sometimes talking can be used as a smokescreen to hide feelings, but silence often forces a person to confront him- or herself and to experience feelings.

Four kinds of silences occur in the counseling relationship. It is critical for the counselor to be able to recognize the kind and quality of each silence.

The Embarrassed Silence

The embarrassed silence usually occurs early in the interaction; the client is expecting the counselor to act and fill the void, but the counselor doesn't. The counselor must not break this silence. This is the empowering, mobilizing silence: The discomfort generated in the client becomes a powerful motivator for client action. A parent in one of my counseling groups once said to me,

I get the feeling sometimes as though there is a big lump of time out there on the table, and when it gets silent, it just fritters away and I get very anxious. At times I get angry at you for not speaking and telling me things. I realize now that if I want something to happen here, I have to act, and that is a good thing for me.

Embarrassed silences diminish almost to nothing over the life span of the relationship.

Changing-Topic Silence

The changing-topic silence occurs in groups and in one-on-one counseling when the individuals reflect on whether they have more to say on the topic at hand. The counselor can use the silence to introduce a topic, although it is best to do that after enough silences have occurred so that the group or individual realizes that the counselor is not taking the responsibility for filling the silence. Generally I find that if I have a topic of concern, I bring this up at the meeting's start. This clears my head so I am able to listen rather than wait for a chance to introduce my topic.

The Reflective Silence

The reflective silence invariably follows some emotionally laden material. This silence is a time-out for thinking about and experiencing the feelings that have been brought to the surface. The reflective silence—a very heavy, palpable feeling—takes a great effort to break. I think the deepest feelings take place in silence, and I think all of the really important work is done in silence. I like the Michel de Montaigne quote that "A bore is someone who takes my solitude and gives me nothing in return." I always relish the companionship of a thoughtful silence. Group meetings very often end on this silence, and the feelings generated by it are discussed on another day.

The Termination Silence

Sometimes a client or group lapses into a silence toward the end of a session that has the quality of the changing-topic silence, except that the group or individual is tired and the work for that day is done. Occasionally I have misinterpreted the termination silence and thought it was the pause before a new topic was to be introduced. I have learned now to check with groups when this happens to determine if they are finished.

Contracting

In contracting—a technique used extensively in the behavioral approach—the assumptions underlying the clinician–client relationship are made explicit. The client is required to be explicit about what is wanted from the clinician, and the clinician has to be explicit about what will or will not be done for the client. Initial sessions are devoted almost solely to the contracting issue. Periodically, as the relationship progresses, time is taken to renegotiate the contract, if needed.

I find it very important to delineate carefully what I expect from clients. Many relationships fail because of expectations that are implicit and not complementary. For example, clients who expect the therapist to rescue them and are working with a therapist who expects the clients to be very active will have a difficult time unless they can negotiate the differences. If the clients and therapist do not deal with this issue, the relationship will deteriorate and anger will develop, although it probably will be directed at an inappropriate source.

Basically, a contract specifies how long the relationship will last, what it will entail, and what the purpose is. Contracts do not have to be detailed or legalistic, but they have to be understood by everybody involved. In particular, I think the time issue needs to be very clear. Before I start a session, I am always explicit about how much time I have in a given encounter, and I am very rigid about terminating when I said I would. I very seldom extend a session beyond the contracted time. The limited time then serves as an impetus (death awareness) to the clients to work toward solving their problems. If I had an open-ended commitment, clients would tend to avoid dealing with painful material, thinking that they could get to it at some vague future date. It is no accident that more affect-laden material is revealed at the session's end than at its beginning.

I remain open to renegotiating contracts. As relationships change, needs change. I never unilaterally change a relationship; it has to be discussed and agreed on. Sometimes neither the client nor I can arrive at a mutually satisfactory contract. When this happens, we terminate. I generally refer the client (if he or she desires) to someone whom I think can meet the client's needs. I usually make more than one referral so the client has a choice. I have ceased trying to be all things to all people, and I recognize that there are some people I cannot help or, more accurately, choose not to help because to do so would violate my personal values. Invariably, the irresolvable issue is responsibility assumption, where the client persistently wants me to do much more than I think is prudent for effecting growth.

Counselor Feedback

The counselor's feelings about a client should be judiciously shared with him or her. Although this sharing can facilitate client growth, it must always be done within a context of support, and the timing must be precise. For example, one participant in a student clinician group was especially verbose and continually repeated herself. Toward the end of one of her monologues, I interrupted and commented, "Anne, I find your initial statements and thoughts very interesting, but when you keep repeating yourself, I find myself getting bored and emotionally distanced from you." The comment encouraged her to begin talking about how other people had given her similar feedback and that her verbosity reflected her loneliness and insecurity. The rest of the group, which up to that point had been sitting with glazed-over eyes, began to give her more feedback. The result was a fruitful discussion of loneliness and the things people sometimes do that distance other people.

When feedback is given, it is important that the person who delivers the feedback comment about his or her own feelings. In the example I just gave, I did not say, "You talk too much," which would have put her on the defensive. I spoke only about what was going on in my mind. As presented, the problem was mine, not hers, and as long as I talk about myself, I am always an expert.

Counseling Effectiveness

A frequent mistake made by the neophyte counselor is thinking that the goal of counseling is to eliminate the client's pain. This idea is natural in a helping profession; however, it is not healthy to take responsibility for another's pain. By trying to make the person feel better, the clinician often invalidates the client. It is seldom useful to say or imply that a person should not feel emotional pain because it generally causes people to feel guilty.

It is so easy to learn to not express our painful feelings because doing so imposes pain on others. My grandson, who is 4 years old, was recently left in my care for several days. On the first day we went to a playground and a zoo and had lunch at a fast-food restaurant. At home we watched *The Lion King* and played the game Candyland. After his bedtime story, when both exhausted grandfather and exhausted grandson were ready for bed, he said, "I miss my mommy and daddy." Threatened grandfather then responded: "Look at all the nice things we did today," which also said to him that he had no right to feel the way he did and that an honest expressions of his feelings was painful to me. I should have said, "You must love them very much," but I did not find it at the time—only after I had reflected about what had happened.

Emotional pain in a person with a communication disorder is normal. I expect people to feel sad when bad things happen to them; if I do not encounter pain in people who have a communication disorder or in their families, I wonder how they are dealing with this catastrophe. A mother of a child who had just been diagnosed as deaf told me that she was "doing this badly" because she was crying for several hours every day. I assured her that she was not doing badly but was reacting normally. Professionals can be most helpful to their clients by eliminating the negative feelings about the pain that they are experiencing; however, we cannot take away the pain. A core level of pain will remain in any permanent disability. The goal of counseling is to detach the feelings from self-defeating behavior. I try never to judge feelings; they simply exist and I accept them. I can, however, work with clients on what constitutes constructive behavior. Thus, a parent who says, "I can feel guilty and I can still act in a way that is in my own and my child's best interest" has grown successfully. Over time and with careful professional attention, clients find that feelings no longer control them, and "guilty" parents find that they do not have to overprotect their children. Client behavior has to be the ultimate criterion by which we judge the effectiveness of counseling. With time and help, the feelings transform into productive behavior. The anger becomes the energy to make changes; the guilt becomes commitment. Confusion becomes the spur to learning and vulnerability becomes the impetus to reshuffle values. The pain becomes a soft melancholy that intensifies all other feelings.

Professional Humility

If one is to counsel from a humanistic frame of reference—to accept and not prescribe—then one must learn professional humility. Fortunately for me, this occurred rather early in my counseling career. My first clinical experiences stayed with me as though imprinted. Nearly 40 years later, I can still recall the following experience vividly.

Johnny was a 2-year-old child with a hearing impairment in the Emerson College nursery group. He would enter the nursery with his thumb in his mouth and his little finger stuck up one nostril. The finger stayed in his nostril the whole two hours of the nursery day, which included 30 minutes of individual speech–language therapy. It was rather hard to relate to someone with his thumb in his mouth and almost impossible for the child to speak. Johnny never participated in nursery activities, preferring to watch the other children. The staff became convinced that he was emotionally disturbed. One goal of the therapy was to condition Johnny to remove his thumb from his mouth; another goal was to get Johnny's parents to seek psychiatric help. I assumed the latter responsibility, sitting next to his mother during nursery activities and during speech therapy and pointing out to her how deficient Johnny was in comparison with the other children.

The mother refused to see any of the nonparticipatory behavior as abnormal, and she always seemed to have an explanation for his behavior. Consequently, the clinic was unsuccessful on both counts: The thumb remained in the child's mouth until the end of the semester, and the parents decided, much to our dismay and over our objections, to put Johnny in a hearing nursery school and provide him with individual speech and language therapy. The parents left the program. Several months later, I chanced to meet the father socially and of course wanted to know how Johnny was doing. He told me with a big smile on his face, "Johnny kissed his teacher." Well, I thought, at least they got his hand out of his mouth—or did they? The family moved to the West Coast, and as often happens in this business, we lost all contact.

Several years later I happened to be at a meeting on the West Coast and met Johnny's mother. (She had decided to become a speech–language pathologist.) She came armed with all his school records, and I found out that Johnny was attending his neighborhood school, fully mainstreamed, and—as shown by his recent achievement test—was operating at grade level and demonstrating normal social skills.

Fortunately, this family had enough strength to resist my manipulation. I often think of this case and wonder how many of my early prognostications were far off the mark; I suspect a great many. The professional does not have access to all the relevant data. The parent or client knows much more of the really important data for making life decisions, and although at times it has been painful to my professional ego, I have learned to trust people to make their own decisions. I figure that they know what is best for themselves.

Humility helps the counselor develop listening skills. Once the counselor recognizes his or her own limitations, he or she can put aside the personal point of view about what the client should do. If we as counselors have a point of view, then listening stops; we listen only for the weakness so as to present our arguments and thus have our point of view prevail. I did not hear Johnny's mother; I thought only that this was a mother who was denying that she had a child with multiple problems, and I filtered everything she said through that perception. I did not respond to her concerns or fears or credit her content; instead, we were engaged in an adversarial relationship that did not grow and—more important—did not benefit her child.

Counselor Mistakes

I have made mistakes on many occasions. Usually these errors are not so much failures of commission as failures to capitalize on a very cogent situation. I almost always recover from my insensitivities and gaffes. I bring them up at the next session, or if I am really bothered by them, I call up the client and apologize. These apologies have helped relationships because they convey my humanity and my vulnerability, both of which contribute to client growth.

The failure to capitalize on situations, however, is a reflection on my lack of skill at the time. I cannot guarantee to clients that I will always be skillful. I can only promise that I will be doing the best I know how to do at that time and will continue to be a learning and growing professional. I am certainly a better clinician now than I was 10 years ago, and if I last another 10 years, not as good as I will be. I can only give to clients the best of what I have at that time.

I have observers in the form of practicum students in all my parent groups. After each session, we conduct a "postmortem" with an eye to what I might have done differently. I find these sessions very helpful, and many times I can recover from a mistake, although it is never quite the same as having acted a certain way initially. These are the "should have dones" that I think all professionals carry with them. Early in my career I tape-recorded sessions and listened carefully to the playbacks, which helped me identify areas on which I needed to work. In more than 40 years of doing this, I still find those areas. This keeps me going because I always feel professionally challenged. I guess when I finally do it all right all the time, it will be time for me to retire for good.

The Unattractive Client

Occasionally I meet a client toward whom it is difficult to develop an unconditionally positive regard. These clients are like weeds in the garden and bring to mind the Ralph Waldo Emerson quote, "A weed is a plant whose virtues have not yet been discovered." I have to keep searching with these "weeds" to find those virtues. I have found that with care and patience, some of my ugliest weeds have turned into beautiful flowers. Unfortunately, some have remained weeds. If I cannot see them as weeds looking for a place to belong, then I try to see them as teachers, which usually works.

Counseling Caveats

As mentioned in the introduction, effective counseling is often as much a matter of what you don't do as what you actually do. The following is a list of some common pitfalls.

Stereotyping

Stereotyping is a seemingly efficient way of viewing people by putting them into "little boxes" of characteristics. If we do this long enough, we cease to see who is actually there and respond only to our expectations of them. I strenuously avoid reading any material that purports to describe the characteristics of a cultural minority because it invariably leads to cultural stereotyping. In my experience, no two women, no two African Americans, no two Jews, and no two Hispanics are exactly alike. This is especially true for parents of children with special needs. They respond in many different ways to their child's disabilities, and I must put aside my preconceptions when I encounter a new family. For example, some parents are cognitively focused and need a great deal of content initially in order to feel secure, despite what I have frequently stated in this text. This is why it is essential to listen carefully to each client at the outset in order to be truly culturally sensitive and effective; the client will teach us how best to help him or her. Each client must be viewed as a marvelous experiment of one: we are all multicultural.

Transference

Transference occurs whenever we bring our prior learning experiences into the present. Whenever I respond intensely to someone at a first meeting, this is a red flag for me. Because I have had no prior history with that person, I am responding from an imprinting that occurred in my past. For example, I tend to give 10 IQ points to any man who has a mustache like my father's—usually much to my dismay. These kinds of transferences can lead us astray in our dealings with clients because, here again, we cease to see the client or person and respond to the person of whom they remind us. I have found, as I have gotten older, and maybe wiser, that I seem to have less transferences. I think that with age my early life experiences have less influence on my current perceptions. As we get older, we can free ourselves from our past and reinvent ourselves, which I find encouraging.

Projection

Projection closely resembles transference in that we are putting our issues onto the client. In transference it is our past; in projection, it is our current issues and values. It is often very difficult to see our projections. For example, I frequently get asked by a speech and hearing professional about when I refer a client for counseling. I usually respond with the counterquestion "Who has the problem here?" We then generally arrive at the conclusion that it is the professional who has the problem, which is based on his or her fear of entering into the affect realm with the client. It is very easy to project our insecurities onto our clients. Another projection question I frequently get asked is "How do you get fathers to attend the nursery?" The answer is, we don't. Some families work quite well without us ever seeing the father, with both parents quite happy in their roles. We need to take families as they come, not as we would like them to be. Projections always lead to a judgmental attitude that will limit severely the ability to counsel. Whenever we begin thinking that someone else *should* do something, it is a marker of a projection. What the "should" means is that we would do that in that situation, but it does not necessarily mean that it would be good for that person. We need to abandon our egocentric view of the world and accept people as they are. When we do that, they can grow.

Implicit Expectations

Probably nothing damages relationships more than implicit expectations, which are the assumptions we make about the other person's obligations without bothering to explicitly contract for them. This occurs frequently in parent–professional relationships around the subject of responsibility assumption. Parents often enter into the relationship expecting the therapist to "fix" the problem; after all, they are paying for his or her services. The professional, on the other hand, has an expectation that the parents will participate fully in the therapy and that his or her role is to coach and support them. If these conflicting assumptions are not made explicit and negotiated, the relationship will founder. At the outset, the therapist needs to elicit from the client his or her expectations of the relationship and then clarify what can be offered. If no match can be found, then a referral needs to be made. I have had to learn—painfully at times—that I can't help everybody and that it is best to accept clients whose expectations are within my clinical limitations.

Overhelping

This caveat was described earlier as the Annie Sullivan syndrome. If we assume too much responsibility for the clinical outcome, we can inadvertently teach our clients to be helpless. The more we help people overtly, the less they do and the fewer opportunities they have to develop their own resources. We give to life what life demands of us. In many instances, adversity is our best teacher because it forces us to develop capacities that might otherwise lie dormant. Clinicians must find the therapeutic "equator" for helping each family. We must be gentle coaches, helping as covertly as possible and allowing families to take full credit for their successes. Some families will require little assistance, others will require much more. As good teachers, we want to be operating on the periphery of what the families are ready to master, armed always with the assumption and attitude that they are competent individuals. Our goal is to empower, and we do this best not by overhelping but by being there in a supportive way. Finding the appropriate entry point for counseling for each family is what distinguishes the superior clinician from the mediocre one.

Denial Misunderstood

This has already been noted and will be discussed in more detail in the next chapter, but it bears repeating here because failure to appreciate denial frequently confounds the client–professional relationship. When clinicians do not understand the role denial plays in the client's life, an adversarial relationship usually develops. Denial is an emotion-based form of coping derived from the client's fears. It seems to the insensitive clinician that the client or the family is not following through with good recommendations, which usually generates anger on the part of the clinician. The clinician needs to look deeper into the client's or family's behavior. People cannot be pushed out of denial because doing so will only lead to passive-aggressive behavior and a subtle or not-so-subtle adversarial relationship will develop, which will not be helpful. To take denial away would be cruel and generally futile. When client's confidence is high, then denial can be given up and other more fruitful forms of coping can be developed. Therapeutic attention needs to be directed towards building self-esteem and then denial will disappear.

Cheerleading

As helping professionals, our instincts are to take away pain. This is a good and natural tendency that led many of us to select a helping profession in the first place. However, this instinct is not always helpful to our clients. As mentioned in the first chapter, cheering up people in pain only serves to invalidate their feelings. We are telling them that they have no right to their feelings. As such, this only serves to make them feel guilty because they are in pain. With all communication disorders there is a core level of pain that cannot be altered; it needs acknowledgement and acceptance. What our clients need most is to be listened to and have their feelings acknowledged and validated.

The following anonymously written piece says it all about counseling:

> When I ask you to listen to me and you start giving advice, you have not
>   done what I asked.
> When I ask you to listen to me
> and you begin to tell me why I shouldn't feel that way, you are
>   trampling on my feelings.
> When I ask you to listen to me
> and you feel you have to do something to solve my problem, you have
>   failed me, strange as that may seem.
> Listen! All I asked was that you listen.
> Not talk or do—just hear me.
> Advice is cheap: 10 cents will get you both Dear Abby and Billy
>   Graham in the same newspaper.
> And I can do for myself; I'm not helpless.
> Maybe discouraged and faltering, but not helpless.
> When you do something for me that I can and need to do for myself,
>   you contribute to my fear and weakness.
> But when you accept as a simple fact that I do feel what I feel, no
>   matter how irrational, then I can quit trying to convince you and
>   can get about the business of understanding what's behind this
>   irrational feeling. And when that's clear, the answers are obvious
>   and I don't need advice.

Irrational feelings make sense when we understand what's behind them. Perhaps that's why prayer works, sometimes, for some people because, as the poem goes on to say,

> God is mute, and He doesn't give advice or try to fix things. "They" just
>   listen and let you work it out for yourself.
> So, please listen and just hear me. And, if you want to talk, wait a
>   minute for your turn, and I'll listen to you.

CHAPTER

7

THE GROUP PROCESS

I would like to share my very strong bias in favor of group counseling. I believe that group sessions are a very efficacious way of counseling; in fact, I seldom do formal individual counseling. Within an individual session, I have to be wise and alert; there is no help for me. Within the group setting, many resources are available, and although I act as leader, I do not have to be so all-encompassing. Invariably when I am at a loss, someone in the group rescues me. I think that within a group there is marvelous health, strength, and a collective wisdom that supersedes the wisdom of any one member. The task of the leader is to unleash that wisdom.

My group work has been mainly with parents of children recently diagnosed as having a hearing impairment. I have, however, had experience facilitating other groups: parents of children with other disabilities, adults who are hard of hearing, well family members of the chronically ill, people trying to quit smoking (Sponsored by the American Cancer Society), student clinicians and practicing speech–language pathologists and audiologists. The dynamics of groups are universal and independent of content; however, each group is unique and always presents a clinical challenge.

Groups in Speech–Language Pathology and Audiology

It is difficult to determine from the literature on communication disorders just how extensively groups are used, but I suspect it is much more frequently than the literature would indicate. Such groups include therapy groups and counseling groups.

117

The therapy group, which is composed of individuals with speech–language disorders, is used fairly frequently, has a long history, and is convened to work on a specific speech or language problem. More than 50 years ago, Backus and Beasley (1951) found that results from group therapy with children with speech disorders were superior to results from individual therapy. Albertini, Smith, and Metz (1983) found that adolescents who are deaf did as well working on their speech within a group as did a control group whose members were receiving individual therapy. In the years between these two reports, many others have been published that support the idea of group therapy (sometimes for no other reason than better use of therapist time). I suspect that many therapy groups are started and maintained in the hope of reducing a therapist's waiting list.

My concern here is the counseling group (not to imply that counseling is not part of a therapy group), which may or may not be composed of individuals who have speech–language disorders. This group has an implicit mandate to deal with feelings. (In practice, I suspect, many counseling groups stay with content because of the therapist's insecurity). The groups are convened and conceived as places where individuals can talk about the feelings generated by having speech–language disabilities or having relatives who have speech–language disabilities. Counseling has been used in a variety of group contexts, such as with parents of children with speech defects (E. Webster, 1968, 1977), parents of deaf children (Dee, 1981), spouses of patients with aphasia (Bardach, 1969; Emerson, 1980), patients who have had a stroke (Singler, 1982), and deaf adults (Schein, 1982). Apparently these groups are used quite frequently, with varying degrees of success, depending on how well the group can overcome the communication problem.

Groups are used extensively outside the field of communication disorders. Seligman (1982) reported on group counseling for special populations, including patients with cancer, people with physical disabilities, older persons, individuals who abuse drugs, prison populations, people with mental retardation, people with visual impairments, and people who have alcoholism. Groups have also been used extensively in dealing with chronic illness (Cole, O'Conner, & Bennett, 1979; Davies, Priddy, & Tinkleberg, 1986; Hinkle, 1991; McKelvey & Borgerson, 1990). Nuland (1994) underscored the healing properties of groups for the families of people with Alzheimer's disease:

> In the case of Alzheimer's disease, it is rarely the patient who recognizes the need for company in the journey through travail. But there is probably no disability of our time in which the presence of support groups can help so decisively to ensure the emotional survival of the closest witness to the disintegration. . . . There is strength in numbers, even when the numbers

are only one or two understanding people who can soften the anguish by the simple act of listening. (p. 106)

Probably the most extensive use of group techniques has been in the field of psychotherapy. The definitive text in group psychotherapy to date was written by Yalom (1975), who identified 11 interdependent curative factors in group therapy. I think that eight of these factors (which are described in the next section) have wide applicability in counseling groups within the communication disorders field. (I believe that the three other curative factors that Yalom listed—the development of socialization techniques, imitative behavior, and the corrective recapitulation of the primary family group—either are contained within the other factors or are more appropriate for psychotherapeutic groups.)

Curative Factors in Groups

Instillation of Hope

I have an almost mystical belief in the power of the group for healing and growth. By seeing how others have improved or coped with the problem, the client can feel hope for him- or herself. This is something that only clients can give to each other. There is always someone in a group who has overcome adversity, which lifts the spirits of the others. In fact, faith and hope may be the only curative factors one needs, as evidenced by the efficacy of faith healers and placebo therapy. The faith of the therapist in the group process is also transmitted to the clients.

Universality

The group helps individuals recognize that they are not alone in their feelings and perceptions. Parents of a child with a disability often feel that they are crazy or sick for feeling a particular way (which usually involves wishing the child were dead), and when they find out that other parents have felt the same way, they feel relieved. They are not alone, and they are not crazy. Universality—a feeling that you can get only within a group format—is very much a factor in dealing with the existential issue of loneliness.

Imparting of Information

Information is provided not only by the leader, although many groups are structured so that the leader provides most of the content, but also by the other members of the group. I am always astonished at how much clients already know. Sometimes some of the least articulate members in the group come up with marvelous, unique solutions. This is also a primary means of building self-esteem and thus empowering the participants if the facilitator is willing to let the group members be smart. I am also struck by how rarely advice is directly beneficial to a group member, although it is frequently offered within the group. I believe that advice is the indirect conveyance of a mutual interest and caring and as such serves a vital function in the group. Of much more lasting value, however, is the knowledge gained from the sharing of experiences. All groups should and almost always do leave the participants more informed than when the group started.

Altruism

By imparting information, group participants get a chance to help one another. People with disabilities rarely have the chance to help anyone, which diminishes their self-esteem. The group situation enables them to receive help without a concomitant loss of self-esteem because the help is reciprocal.

Within the group, members offer support, reassurance, and insights to one another. I have found, for example, that parents of children with disabilities listen much more attentively to another parent than they do to me. Another parent has a credibility that I can never duplicate. A frequent result of a successful counseling group is the desire—and the translation of that desire into action—to help other persons with similar disabilities. This is a healthy result that has the potential to (a) move the participants away from an almost morbid self-absorption and (b) allow them to grow.

Interpersonal Learning

Human survival depends on the ability to live in groups; yet, I find that many people with whom I come in contact (parents of children with disabilities, student clinicians, speech–language pathologists, audiologists) have poor interpersonal skills. I think this is due in part to poor early learning in their family of origin. They have difficulty communicating with others, being trusting and honest with others, and learning to love more fully. None of this is pathological in the sense that these people are nonfunctional; however, better developed interpersonal skills would enable them to get more joy and satisfaction out of all of their interpersonal interactions. The group can be a safe vehicle for the participants to enhance their interpersonal learning. They can learn (or more appropriately relearn) how to be more open and accepting of others and can then take this knowledge from the group context into other relationships.

Group Cohesiveness

Cohesiveness, a basic property of groups, is difficult to define and grasp, but I think it is an integral factor in successful counseling. Analogous to the relationship in individual therapy, cohesiveness is not a curative factor per se but rather a precondition. Cohesiveness is related to the attractiveness of the group to its members. I know a group will be successful when I can hardly wait for the sessions to start and I look forward to seeing the other members of the group. Cohesiveness is intricately tied to trust: Where trust develops, as in individual therapy, groups come together and growth can occur. Whenever someone in a group reveals a deep secret that is accepted and amplified by other members of the group, there is a quantum leap in group cohesiveness.

Another intangible factor, an interpersonal attraction that may or may not occur, also determines cohesiveness. Some groups seem to come together very easily, and I do not have to work for cohesiveness. The members of these groups are attracted to one another because of similar values and, I suspect, because of some transferences that they bring to the experience. The chemistry in these groups seems right; there is a good mix of talkers and listeners, and individuals like each other. You can not predict cohesiveness in advance. It is something that develops over time. In other groups, cohesiveness is hard to come by— members do not especially like each other or share much. I tend to want to blame the lack of cohesiveness on bad group chemistry and not on my lack of skill. When pressed to the wall, however, I admit a skill issue: I need to pay more careful attention to building trust and cohesiveness in the early stages with groups and to quickly identify when a group is not developing them.

Although I think individuals can and do learn even when a group is not cohesive, I think that the learning is greater and much deeper in a cohesive group. Many of my lifelong and close friendships have developed from being in groups with high degrees of cohesiveness.

Catharsis

Catharsis, which is closely related to universality, is the expression of the considerable affect that surrounds communication disorders. Almost all participants bring to the group pent-up emotions that they have had no safe place to express. The group can provide the vehicle for the release and sharing of these feelings. Families of patients who have had strokes, for example, invariably come to feel that they can talk in the group because they can be understood. Professional groups tend to bring individuals' feelings of inadequacy to the fore, and there is a great deal of relief in being able to express them and to be heard and understood by the other group members.

Catharsis per se is not a curative factor; simply expressing a feeling is not sufficient to promote growth. It is, however, a preliminary to being able to unhook the feelings from the unhealthy behavior.

Existential Issues

Existential issues are described in detail in Chapter 2. Groups give individuals a chance to work through their questions regarding the issues of death and life enhancement, responsibility assumption and dependency, loneliness and love, and meaninglessness and commitment. Almost all of the personal growth that emerges in the groups I facilitate emerges around the existential issues. They are a powerful way of looking at individuals and judging personal growth. When groups, and the individuals within groups, are willing to face the existential issues, growth and change begin.

Group Goals in Communication Disorders

Yalom's (1975) 11 factors can all be subsumed under three broad categories that relate to groups within the field of communication disorders: conveying content, sharing of affect, and realizing personal growth. The goals are contained within the curative factors and need only be discussed briefly as they relate to communication disorders.

Content

All groups to a certain extent have a content mandate; that is, the convening of the group makes possible the sharing of information and experiences of the members. Learning is unavoidable within a group context, although sometimes what is learned is what the leader neither expected nor intended. Groups proceed best when the leader is not perceived as the sole source of content. This may violate group members' expectations at first, but in the long run, more is learned from the group experience when there is a collective responsibility to teach one another. Unfortunately, many groups within the field of communication disorders seem to have content dissemination as their sole purpose, and usually this content is supplied by the professional. These groups are missing out on a lot.

Affect Release

Being the parent of a child with a disability, having an important family member undergo a catastrophic illness, or having a communication disorder will engender a great many feelings that usually have no healthy way of being expressed. Frequently the person's feelings, especially anger, are repressed, which results in depression, or are displaced to others, which impairs interpersonal relationships. The group can become the means for releasing the affect in a safe environment among people who understand those feelings. More than any other vehicle I know, the group can give sanction and permission to its members to experience their feelings. It is absolutely essential that the group leader establish a norm that feelings just *are* and as such must never be judged. Without this norm firmly in place, no group will ever develop the intimacy and cohesiveness that promotes maximum growth.

Personal Growth

Personal growth is not ordinarily thought of as a responsibility within the discipline of communication disorders, yet I believe that we must address this issue in order to be more effective as professionals. For example, we need to help parents of children with disabilities become more assertive and less compliant when participating with professionals in making educational plans for their child. For this to happen, the parents (as well as all people with communication disorders) need to have high self-esteem and a more internal locus of control. People with communication disorders have to learn to take responsibility for their disabilities in order to minimize the negative effects on their personal lives. They may learn ways of using their disorder to help others, such as when they form self-help and political action groups to further benefit persons with disabilities in our society. A group can serve as a powerful personal growth vehicle by allowing individuals to help others, and if the leader is willing to "sit on" his or her wisdom, the group members can take control and therefore learn responsibility assumption. This cannot help but carry over into their everyday lives.

Principles of Group Functioning

Leadership

The leadership of the group is a vital factor in determining its success. Groups are entities unto themselves; that is, each group has a unique personality and no two groups are ever the same. The principles underlying successful individual counseling are equally applicable to counseling within a group setting. The counselor must treat the group from a humanistic point of view, with acceptance, genuineness, empathy, and concern. The leader must be seen as a caring person. In his exhaustive study of encounter groups, Yalom (1975) found four leadership functions that were directly related to outcomes:

1. *Emotional stimulation*—accomplished by confronting, modeling, risk-taking, and disclosing self.
2. *Caring*—accomplished by offering support, affection, warmth, concern, and genuineness.
3. *Meaning attribution*—accomplished by exploring, clarifying, interpreting, and providing a cognitive framework for change.
4. *Executive function*—accomplished by setting limits and rules, managing time, and suggesting procedures. (p. 477)

Lieberman, Yalom, and Miles (1973) found that (a) those leaders who were very high in caring and meaning attribution and who were moderate in emotional stimulation and executive function were the most successful, and (b) their successes were independent of their theoretical orientations. Group members grew with leaders who cared about them and could give them a cognitive framework for understanding their behavior. Groups were limited in their growth by leaders who were too high or too low in provoking feelings and in executive function. Too little executive function tended to create confused groups, whereas too much tended to create passive ones. Too little emotional stimulation led to devitalized groups, whereas emotionally overcharged groups were chaotic.

In my experience with parent and caregiver groups in particular, I have found that it is seldom necessary to provide emotional stimulation. The affect is so high to begin with that by providing a safe, caring atmosphere, I allow the feelings to emerge without any need to provoke them.

Establishment of Group Norms

The most important function of the leader is to set norms for the group. These are the implicit and sometimes very explicit rules by which the group is to function. A group's norms are established very early and are hard to change once established. The leader establishes these norms by modeling and, especially with procedural norms, by explicitly stating them. The most frequently used mechanism for establishing norms in the group is the reinforcement paradigm. By virtue of the power accorded to him or her by the members of the group, the leader uses social approval as a powerful reinforcement agent to ensure group norms. As a result, those behaviors or remarks chosen to be acknowledged tend to become valued by the group, and those behaviors that are not acknowledged tend to be devalued. Most leaders reinforce norms unwittingly, based on some deep-seated and unconscious prejudices that they have.

I think my greatest source of failure with groups has been in allowing unhealthy group norms to develop and in not acting soon enough to prevent a poor norm from taking hold. In one group that I was leading, I was called away to answer the phone (something I no longer allow to happen), and when I returned, the parents were having a passionate discussion concerning which was the best diaper to use on their children. I listened for a while and then very stupidly confronted the group as to why they were wasting their group time discussing such a trivial topic when they could do that elsewhere. The group thereafter became a very low-risk, low-contributing group, one of the dullest groups with which I ever worked. When I was finally able to see what was happening (2 months later—I can be a bit slow), I realized that I had established a norm of leader-generated topics. Apparently, as far as the group was concerned, only certain topics were appropriate to discuss within the meeting, and they had to guess what was acceptable because if they did not, they would incur my wrath. The best strategy for them to adopt was to play it safe and not take a risk by trying to introduce a new topic. The topics groups select to discuss are never irrelevant; however, leaders sometimes are.

This group never recovered. If I had it to do over again (a lament most professionals share), I would say, "It must be so hard for you when you have so many choices." This remark might have moved the group to look at all the choices they had to make regarding their children. At the very least, I would have done better to have kept quiet and allowed some other members to point out how they were wasting time. In either case, I do not think that I would have had a dull group.

Interactional Norm

If group members are to relate and learn from one another, they have to interact among themselves. Most groups begin with a question directed toward the leader. If the question is answered, another question-and-answer exchange is usually encouraged. This means that the leader can get trapped into providing content via answering the questions and speaking about 50% of the time. If the group is to function as a group, the leader has to quickly get away from answering questions and encourage interactions among all the group members. I have observed groups that are basically individual therapies within a group setting. I don't feel these are as productive as when the members interact with each other.

If I take up no more than 10% of the group's time by talking, it usually becomes a successful group. The interactional norm allows for the sharing of information and for the helping that can occur among members.

Initiative Norm

I think the initiative norm is vital for growth: The group members must learn that if they want something to happen, they must make it happen. I come into the group with no agenda and no list of topics. The topics will be determined by the group, and if they wish to sit and be passive, nothing happens. Early in the history of a group, a silence descends while the group waits to be told what to do and how to proceed. If the leader takes control at this juncture, the norm of a leader-controlled group is established. Once this happens, the members become spectators, and the leader can become very resentful about doing all the work. It is very hard for a professional to not take the initiative because it conforms to the implicit expectations of both the professional and the clients. This must be resisted, and is was the hardest thing for me to learn at the beginning of my work with groups. It relates to wanting to rescue a group from its felt inadequacies. I almost never use structured experiences early in the life of a group because that also establishes a leader-initiated group.

Self-Disclosure

Self-disclosure is a necessary component of growth. It is hard for me to see how group participants can learn if they are unwilling to share themselves. I must establish a group norm whereby when individuals do reveal something, they are never penalized and are always supported. Self-disclosure must always be safe, especially when a participant finally reveals his or her "guilty secret." A parent group will become very cohesive when another parent can say, "I always felt that way," or when other members will accept the secret without saying or implying that the group member should not feel that way. When there are many "shoulds" floating around, groups become inhibited and little self-disclosure occurs.

In one group I facilitated, a man with a laryngectomy revealed for the first time that he never used his artificial larynx when he went outside because it embarrassed him. None of the other group members told him that he "should" use his larynx; instead, they listened and expressed to him their understanding of how hard it was to appear so deviant. After a while, he began crying and received a great deal of emotional support from the group. Several sessions later, he announced that he was now using the larynx in public.

Self-disclosure should never be forced. Participants need to feel free to not reveal themselves if they so desire (which is actually another norm in itself).

One way that the leader can encourage self-disclosure is by revealing something about him- or herself, which can be tricky because the timing must be precise. Early in the group's life, an important issue is the leader's credibility. If the leader's vulnerabilities are revealed too soon, that credibility may be sacrificed. Self-disclosure by the leader can be very helpful for the group because it helps dispel the authority issue. Clients can see that professionals are human and sometimes need the help that the group can provide. I am, however, very reluctant to self-disclose too early in the life of the group, and I expect that the self-disclosure norm will develop spontaneously from the emotional need for validation and from the trust and acceptance norms that begin to develop.

Confrontation

It is vital that group members learn to "check out" with one another when they are concerned about something. Many problems in interpersonal relationships occur from making assumptions without any checks on reality. For example, a student who assumed I was angry with her because I did not smile when we met could operate on that assumption to the detriment of our relationship. If, however, we had established a confrontation norm, the student would feel free to question me on how I felt about her and might find that I had been preoccupied with some personal problems and that my not smiling was not a reflection of how I felt about her. If in fact I was angry with her, then we would have an opportunity to discuss what was interfering with our relationship. In either event, we would both win from the confrontation and our relationship could then develop further. I can relax in a group once a confrontation norm has been established because it means that my behavior and statements will not be misunderstood or go unquestioned: The participants will test reality with me and with each other if needed.

The confrontation norm is best established by role modeling, and the leader must select an appropriate time to demonstrate this behavior. Confrontation requires a great deal of group trust and is frightening to members. Unfortunately, this norm is not common in many interpersonal relationships, and participants are usually fearful when confrontations occur. Confrontation is closely related to self-disclosure because all confrontation involves a disclosure of self in regard to another person. Self-disclosure generally emerges first because it is safer to talk only about oneself than it is to talk about oneself in relation to someone else who is present. The same conditions that lead a group to self-disclosure also lead to developing a confrontation norm.

Confrontation is not necessarily about negative feelings to one can also confront others with feelings of warmth and liking. I find, however, that the first confrontation feelings to emerge are very often anger and resentment. Unfortunately, most people are less threatened by expressing angry feelings than they are by expressing loving feelings.

Here-and-Now Norm

Probably nothing is deadlier in a group than having members tell long anecdotes to which nobody else has access; interest in the group diminishes rapidly. The facilitator has to find immediacy in the material and bring it to the present. For example, to a participant relating a story in which he had a dispute with the hearing-aid dealer, I might respond, "What did you do with your anger?" (inviting self-disclosure) and then ask, "Have you been angry with me?" (inviting confrontation). The more immediate the experience is, the more exciting it is and the greater the potential for its being a learning experience for everyone. When it is material to which everyone has access, as in recalling an event that happened in one of the group meetings, all the members of the group can contribute, receive, and give feedback.

A here-and-now norm is established by timely interventions on the facilitator's part that force the group member into the present. Groups will not start out with a here-and-now orientation, as they have no history from which to work. Participants have to reveal themselves and establish their credibility. There also needs to be some elapsed time for interactions among members to be processed. Here-and-now is a powerful norm directed toward achieving the goals of personal growth because it encourages interpersonal interaction within the group.

Respecting Individual Needs

Group norms, if not watched, can become very restrictive, especially when they promote a high degree of conformity. It is not healthy for everyone to adhere rigidly to a particular established norm. Individuals need to feel that they have control over their own behaviors and that learning will proceed when they are ready. One of the few explicit norms I establish in every group I lead is that the participants do not have to talk if they do not wish to and that no question must be answered. When a group decision is required, it may be necessary to arrive at a compromise or a willingness of the dissenters to forego their wishes for the good of the group. The back and forth of the negotiations, if done in an atmosphere of mutual respect, is healthy for the group. Greater cohesiveness usually emerges after a successful negotiation.

Procedural Norms

Procedural norms determine how the group will function. There are usually a number of givens over which the group has no control, such as number of sessions and length of time of each session. I am always clear at the outset about how much time is available. If time is a negotiable issue with the group, I enter into negotiation at the first session so that everyone knows the length of their time commitment and agrees to it. I also am sure to be at the group meetings on time and to end all meetings at the agreed-upon hour.

I try to establish a norm of confidentiality in almost all counseling groups that I lead. I know I cannot impose confidentiality because I have no way of enforcing it. I tell the group members that I will not talk about them with any outsiders and that I hope they will do the same. I do not allow casual visitors to the group. In my academic classes, I do not talk about confidentiality in initial sessions because confidentiality implies (or almost imposes) a self-disclosure norm on a group. If a group of students begins to self-disclose, I then talk to them about confidentiality and see if we can come to some consensus.

Stages of Group Development

Although each group is unique, all groups seem to develop along similar lines. A group facilitator needs to have a sense of the developmental sequence of groups to be able to diagnose quickly when a group is not functioning and to perhaps provide some corrective measures. Almost invariably the difficulty is caused by an unhealthy group norm that is limiting group growth. Virtually no controlled research studies on group development have been published; those that do exist are mainly nonsystematic clinical observations.

The Group at Inception

I usually start groups by introducing myself, explaining how I came to be there, and stating what expectations I have for myself in the group. I then invite the members to introduce themselves and describe why they are there. After everyone has finished, I mention any procedural norms (i.e., time of sessions, right to not answer questions, and so on). These are kept to a minimum because most norms are developed as a function of how I behave and which group behaviors I will reinforce. I might then remark that I hope that everyone will come to value the experience. Usually at this point a loud silence ensues, which seems to be eternal but is probably no more than 30 seconds in duration. Almost invariably the silence is broken by a question directed at me, which is usually a procedural-type question, as the members begin to look to the leader to provide them with structure. For example, a participant might ask, "What are we supposed to do here?" (I usually respond, "What would you like to do here?")

At inception, the group is primarily engaged in developing structure and establishing credibility. When the members begin to learn that I will not structure the session, they start to act and in doing so reveal themselves. (They also get mad at me for violating their expectations, but this anger seldom emerges in that first session.) Everybody is still on their best "cocktail party" behavior. A parent group might begin with one parent telling a story about discovering her child's disability, which establishes her credentials to be in the group and invariably provokes other members to start telling their stories. When they find nods of acceptance and a matching of experiences, cohesiveness starts to build. Usually a lot of affect is expressed. The beginning stages of a parent group are usually very cathartic as the parents reveal and experience the pent-up feelings that have not previously been expressed.

A student group or a working professional group usually starts out hesitantly with long, embarrassed silences. The members are not sure how to proceed and are uncertain how much of themselves they are willing to reveal. Usually there is someone in the group who is desperate enough to risk some self-disclosure. If that is accepted, an intimacy spiral begins to develop and more and more self-disclosures occur. Professional groups have generally been the most emotionally muted groups with whom I have worked. Often this happens when there is a hierarchical structure to the group such as in groups of students and supervisors or employees and employers; mobilizing these groups requires enormous amounts of patience. These groups may also have a hidden agenda; there is a history of relationships about which the leader has no knowledge, and there are potential traps. Leaders very often are scapegoated by these groups for bringing into the open very painful topics that the group has preferred to ignore.

For example, I once worked with the staff of a school for the deaf. After two very dull sessions punctuated by long silences, the group members began to open up. A great deal of hostility was directed toward one teacher who was chronically late to class and who was not viewed by the other teachers as being very competent. I was able to get them to specify this teacher by not accepting generalizations such as, "Some teachers are always late." I asked them who they had in mind, and when they finally specified one teacher, everyone jumped on the bandwagon. The accused teacher left in a gush of tears. The group then turned on me, and I was accused of causing the problem. The group never became a comfortable place for the members to reveal more about themselves, and it certainly was not a comfortable place for me. I think the group and I learned much from that encounter, and I think the school ultimately benefitted from that teacher's resignation. It is much easier to work with a group of strangers because then the leader is privy to the history of the group from the start, without preconceptions.

A classic dilemma for the group leader occurs when a member of a beginning group is starting to establish destructive norms and nobody is willing to confront him or her. For example, in a recent student group with which I was working, one participant kept monopolizing the group with long, boring anecdotes that had no relationship to what anyone else had been saying. She filled every silence and commandeered the gaps between silences. Nobody in the group seemed confident enough to challenge her. I took responsibility for pointing out her behavior and solicited feedback from other members as to how they were feeling about her. My intervention came too soon in the group's development because the "monopolizer" started not attending; when she did attend, she seldom spoke. She denied being fearful of speaking but seemed to lose all interest in the group. The rest of the group, however, became even more fearful, afraid that I might put them on the "hot seat." The group became a very low-risk, low-participation group characterized by long, uncomfortable silences and very little self-disclosure. They no longer saw me as a support. Even though I solicited feedback about how they felt about the incident and about me, the group never became cohesive.

In retrospect, I realize that I needed to wait longer before confronting the monopolizer in this group; I did not allow the group time to learn to act cohesively. Groups need time to develop sufficient trust: Familiarity breeds liking when we can get below the surface behavior. I have found it is a mistake to try to push groups in the early stages of development; they operate in an unfolding process. A classic dilemma for the group facilitator is the timing of a confrontation because to wait too long is equally destructive to the group process. In a parent group with which I was working, there was a deaf mother a deaf child. She would not let the other mothers grieve about their children's deafness. Every time they tried to say something negative about deafness, the woman would say, "But look at me," meaning that she was functioning as a wife and mother and had made a good adjustment to her deafness. However, the other parents were only seeing that her speech was virtually unintelligible and that she needed an interpreter to function in the group; they were still very much in the denial and resistance stages of coping. It was a problem that I never really resolved. The group was very restricted, and its members needed to be confronted by the group leader, but I never found what seemed to me a satisfactory time to confront them. I think I lacked the professional courage at that time to challenge the group to open up concerning what was happening. This was one of my less successful groups, and I learned much from it. Unfortunately, our clients often suffer when we professionals learn.

Resistance to the group process also begins to develop early. This resistance usually manifests itself by the group members focusing on differences among them. The parent groups that I lead at Emerson College are composed of parents of young children who are deaf, parents of children with normal hearing, student clinicians, and sometimes a practicing clinician who wants to learn more about groups. The professionals and I meet after the group session to process the experience. Almost invariably, the professionals and students participate in the group, at a low level. They feel that it is a parent group and that they have little to contribute. As they become more comfortable, however, they begin to see the commonalities between themselves and the parents, and they frequently use the group as a valuable personal-growth vehicle.

The Working Group

The developmental stages of a group are rarely well demarcated. There is no single point at which a group announces that it is ready to move from the inception stage to the working stage. The latter stage is characterized by cohesiveness, by conflict, and by redefinition of the leader.

It might seem contradictory to say that the group is both cohesive and in conflict, but these attributes are not incompatible. Only when one feels safe within a relationship can one afford to be confrontational. When it emerges within the group, conflict is usually a marker of the level of cohesiveness within the group. In initial stages, everyone is on his or her best behavior, uncertain as to the safety of the situation. When the members feel secure, they confront. Usually the confrontation is with an outsider, as when parents accuse the students of not having a child and therefore not being able to understand them. If no obvious outsider exists, the behavior is usually directed toward the leader for somehow failing them. (The leader in one sense is always an outsider, and acting as group facilitator often means that the leader has to continually confront existential aloneness.)

At this point the group is ready to redefine the leader and settle into its working structure. Anger is directed toward me because I will not tell them what to do, and parents sometimes wonder if I could possibly understand them because I do not have a child with a disability. Conflict cannot be eliminated from human interaction; we grow from it. It is the resolution of conflict that promotes change and growth. We negotiate among ourselves, we compromise, and we develop the mechanisms that enable us to attend to tasks.

Content also becomes very valuable and is readily transferred among the members. A good working group is characterized by a joint knowledge of the strengths and weaknesses of each member and an ability to use the individual talents that are in the group. The topics that appeared in the initial stages of the group now reappear and are discussed in more detail and from different perspectives. Some participants who said little the first time around may become very vocal (the previous discussion may have set them to thinking about the issue when they were not ready to share). Other members may have rethought their positions. I find that with parent groups in particular, all the cogent issues emerge in the first few sessions, and no new topics occur thereafter. Parent groups operate in a recycling manner. A richness and complexity are generated by the interactions of the group members, and they never run out of things to say.

In a well-functioning group, the trust level is high, and when conflict does emerge, it is dealt with openly. Positive feelings among the members emerge, and some are even directed toward the leader, who is now accepted as a working member of the group. I realize I am portraying an idealized vision of the working group. Not all of the groups with which I have dealt achieve this level of functioning, but many get close. I have never failed to learn from a group, and 35 years later, I am still doing it. Maybe when I finally get it right, I will give it up. Groups keep me grounded and are an important component of my own personal growth.

The Terminating Group

Termination is an integral part of the group process and is not to be trivialized or minimized. The process of termination itself becomes an impetus to further growth. My own death-avoidance issues have very often interfered with providing a group with a satisfactory termination ritual. Groups need time and space to tie up loose ends (there are always loose ends) and to mourn their demise. Often the group avoids the task of termination because it is painful. The leader can use that termination awareness as a spur to complete work. I try to keep groups working until the last possible moment. Often groups will start the termination process too soon; if I allow this to happen, some good work can be lost. The leader must exercise judgment concerning timing.

I have terminated groups by suggesting that each member take a moment to reflect on the group experience and to imagine going home. I ask, "What messages do you wish you had delivered? What 'I should have saids' do you think you might have?" I then suggest that we spend the rest of the session delivering the messages. Yalom (1975) said the following about the termination process:

> Throughout, the therapist facilitates the group work by disclosing his own feelings about separation. The therapist, no less than the patients, will miss the group. For him, too, it has been a place of anguish, conflict, fear, and

also of great beauty; some of life's truest and most poignant moments occur in the small and yet limitless microcosm of the therapy group. (p. 374)

Other Considerations

Use of Structured Experiences

Structured experiences are generally any activities, usually generated by the leader, that are designed to accelerate the group process. They are techniques that encourage self-disclosure or bypass the conventional social restrictions. For example, a new group may be divided into dyads in which each member of the dyad interviews the other. When the group reconvenes, each member of the dyad introduces the other person to the group. There are many such devices to help the group through the initial introductory stage.

The problem with leader-directed exercises is that they do not encourage group members to take the initiative. They tend to create a passive group that waits for the leader to give the next exercise. These exercises can become an excuse for an individual's behavior and can limit responsibility assumption. Exercises frequently are used to rescue a group (actually, the leader) and in the long term are seldom helpful. Lieberman et al. (1973) found that group leaders who used exercises most frequently were regarded by the members of their groups as more competent, more effective, and more perceptive than leaders who used structured experiences sparingly; yet, and very much to the point, the members of the highly structured experience groups had the poorest outcomes (i.e., fewer positive changes and less ability to maintain positive change over time) than did the members of the less-structured group.

I have used—and still occasionally use—structured experiences in my work-shops. I use them sparingly, and they need to fit organically within the flow of the group process. When they are effective, they occur or seem to occur sponta-neously. In a previous book (Luterman, 1979), I devoted an entire chapter to structured experience. Structured activities include role playing, hypothetical families (described in the previous chapter), and guided fantasies. Although I have had positive feedback from readers who have used them to advantage, I am always a bit uncomfortable with their use. I feel that these activities can get a group and the group leader into trouble that they may not yet be prepared to handle. Although structured experiences can be valuable if used judiciously, they also can open up members of a group before the group is ready, and they seem to encourage a technique orientation for the group leader that I do not like.

The interested reader is referred to material in my previous book, which can be adapted to any communication disorder.

Homogeneity of Grouping

The general tendency to keep groups homogeneous is usually reflected in the diagnostic label. We have groups of persons with laryngectomies, individuals who stutter, families of patients who have had strokes, and so on. When I began working with groups, I restricted the group to parents of young children who were deaf who otherwise had no problem. I was trying for a very homogeneous group because I did not feel secure enough at that time to handle any additional problems presented by "deviant" parents. I soon learned that homogeneity is a myth. Even though the group shared the same label, there were enormous differences among the group members—differences in education, values, and child-drearing practices. In fact, an early manifestation of resistance to the group process was the pointing out of the many differences that existed among the members (e.g., "They can't possibly understand me because my child is hard of hearing and their children are deaf"). One primary task of the facilitator is to focus the group on their similarities (e.g., by asking, "Can you tell me some ways in which you are like these other people?").

As I have become more secure in my abilities, I have allowed more obviously heterogeneous groupings to occur. I began letting parents of children with multiple disabilities and hearing impairments into the group, parents of older children who are deaf, and parents of children without any hearing problems. Recently, I have worked with groups of parents with children of mixed disabilities. Each time I have increased the apparent heterogeneity of the group, the group has become richer for it. Parents of hearing children have added a commonality to the child rearing problems, parents of older children who are deaf have added their experience, and parents of other children with disabilities have led us to an appreciation of the universality of the experience of parenting a child with a disability. These different parents have stretched me professionally, and I now welcome and encourage diversity in my groups.

Group Size and Setting

Generally, the groups with which I work have between 8 and 15 members. I find that this is a good size because there are enough members for sufficient interactions among the participants but not so many as to require inordinate amounts of time for establishing individuals' credibility. Larger groups take much longer to establish trust. I also do not allow new people to join the group except at clear demarcation points such as semester breaks. New members tend to hold back group development because the group requires time to absorb the newcomer and to reestablish cohesiveness. It also takes time for the new member to figure out the group norms. I have recently broken this "rule" and now allow new parents to enter a working group, although it does present considerable problems to me as the facilitator. I have begun to accept that challenge because I do not want to deny parents the healing properties of the group any longer than necessary.

I always try to hold meetings in a comfortable room and to have the participants sit in a circle so that they and the leader can establish eye contact with each other and can read each other's body language. Chairs also need to be comfortable because most groups meet for 1 to 2 hours. A professor of mine once said that the mind could absorb only as much as the seat can endure.

Filling the Available Time

Group duration is usually arbitrarily determined. The exigencies of calendar, finances, and participant availability seem to have more bearing on group length than does the amount of therapeutic progress. In one sense, groups are never finished; they are always in the process of becoming, and new material is always emerging. In this way, they are not unlike human beings. For me, the group meeting is a magical moment to be enjoyed and savored for that time and never to be replicated.

Groups have a marvelous way of filling the available time. There is a subconscious and collective knowledge as to how far we can go together on our journey. There is an apocryphal story that Carl Rogers was once asked, "How far can you get with nondirective therapy when you have only 20 minutes time?" His reputed response was, "20 minutes worth." I have had some wonderfully intense group experiences that lasted a total of 2 hours. These groups are almost like a speeded-up motion picture: We all knew that we had only 2 hours to work. All the trivialities were eliminated, cohesiveness developed very quickly, and self-disclosure was high. Several of my most satisfying professional experiences have occurred in groups with a very short lifespan.

The counseling group can have a tremendous value in the therapeutic process. It can be used for the families of individuals with communicative disorders as a supplement to individual therapy, or it can be used in conjunction with individual therapy sessions. Groups can be used very flexibly. Developing skills in facilitating groups should be part of a speech–language therapist's training. I think there is no greater gift that we can give to our clients and their families than a well-facilitated support group.

WORKING WITH FAMILIES

Family has always been very important to me. I am part of a second-generation immigrant family; none of my grandparents could speak English very well. Because we were aliens in a strange land, and we were not yet comfortable with the dominant culture, we were forced to rely on each other. My father would frequently tell us children, "Blood is thicker than water," meaning that we could rely on family more then we could on outsiders. When one of us moved, we all moved. I grew up with an extended family of grandparents, aunts, uncles, and cousins all living within 1 mile of each other. From the perspective of 60-odd years, I now see that we were an enmeshed family.

That family injunction of "blood is thicker than water," which is buried deep within my psyche, has carried over to my professional life. After working for several years as a clinical audiologist, I began to feel increasingly uncomfortable with the restricted and limited involvement I had with clients and their families. I remember vividly a clinical experience in which I knew I was "short." (This is another "nugget-of-gold" situation based on sins of omission rather than commission. The clinically short situation is a marker of skills that we are ready to learn but don't quite have yet.) A man about 60 years of age came to me for a hearing aid evaluation. He had recently remarried after spending the previous 5 years as a widower. His new wife was very distressed at his inability to hear and was constantly nagging him to get a hearing aid. He did have an old hearing aid that he had kept in a drawer and wore only occasionally and not very enthusiastically. It was clear from his manner and some of his statements that he was requesting the hearing aid evaluation only at the insistence of his wife, who had not accompanied him to the examination. At that point in my clinical development, I didn't think I had any option but to fulfill the expectations of the client, so I proceeded to test his hearing (he had a steeply sloping audiogram with rather poor speech discrimination) and to try a variety of hearing aids. We found one that was reasonably satisfactory, and I wrote a prescription for the aid (we were not dispensing in those days). My "counseling" consisted of telling him how the aid worked and talking to him about situations in which to use the aid. He never returned for a follow-up visit.

All the time I was testing and counseling him, I knew I needed to be doing something else. This situation demanded a response other than the traditional approach of audiologist as technician. What I realized somewhat later (3 years, to be exact) was that the wife who was not present also had a hearing problem. Because she had a hearing problem, it was my responsibility to help her by including her in the evaluation. If I could have seen this man again, I would have stopped the evaluation at the case history stage and suggested that we set up another appointment so that the wife could be present. At that meeting, having the wife present during the evaluation would have demonstrated to her the limits of his hearing and the limits of amplification for him. We could then have embarked on a discussion of ways to compensate around the home for his reduced acuity. To have included the wife would have been a much more effective clinical strategy then proceeding as I did in treating only the identified patient.

These clinically short situations provide the professional irritant seed that can lead to the development of clinical "pearls." I reaffirmed my prior conviction of how important the family was, and the wisdom that evolved from this less-than-satisfactory clinical encounter led me to develop a family-centered nursery program for young children with hearing impairments. I also insisted from that point on that any clients be accompanied by a family member. I think I became a much more effective clinician, which is the usual result of solving a clinically short situation.

My search to become a more effective clinician led me to the literature in family therapy, which I think is incredibly fruitful for our field and is only now beginning to affect the profession of communication disorders. No one person is credited with developing this area of therapy; instead, the field seems to have developed spontaneously from the work of several disparate clinicians trained to provide individual therapy. Virginia Satir, Salvador Minuchin, Henry Bowen, and Carl Whitaker were forerunners of the current work being done in family therapy (Hoffman, 1981).

At a workshop I attended, Satir told of her introduction to family work. She was a trained psychiatric social worker who had been was assigned to the back wards of a mental hospital. (I have always wondered about the assignments of new teachers and clinicians to the patients or classes that nobody else wants and that all the experienced professionals consider hopeless. I often thought that these classes and clients needed the most experienced clinicians rather than the neophytes, and the system struck me as absurd. But, as I have reflected on it, I have come to the conclusion that perhaps the young clinician does not know that these cases are hopeless and thus gets a better result than the experienced clinician. (Clients have a way of responding to clinician expectations.) Satir found that as her patients who were most problematic were getting better, they were earning weekend passes. When they returned on Monday, she found them more disturbed than when they had left on Friday. She realized that working at the identified patient level was not efficient and began insisting that family members attend the counseling sessions. As these family members began to interact with the identified patient, Satir found that the whole family was dysfunctional and that the patient's illness played a vital role in maintaining the family homeostasis (1967). Very often the identified patient was instrumental in sustaining the parents' marriage by distracting the parents from their marital conflicts. Satir took the whole family in therapy, with excellent results.

Minuchin, Rosman, and Baker (1978) examined families in which children had psychosomatic illnesses. Looking at families of children with asthma, anorexia or diabetes who could not maintain appropriate blood sugar levels, they found almost invariably that in these families the marital relationships were in poor shape and that the children's symptoms were a maintaining factor in the families. The "ill" child in each family had been triangulated into the marital conflict, and the symptoms served to keep the family together, although at a huge cost to the child. If the patients were to get better, the family homeostasis would be threatened, so everyone within the family was invested in keeping the identified patient "sick." Minuchin and other family therapists now direct their clinical energies at the parental level rather than the child level. This approach has yielded highly successful results (Hoffman, 1981).

✻ The basic notion underlying all family therapy is that the family is a system in which all of the components are interdependent. Every family member affects every other component of the family. For the family therapist, there is no such thing as individual therapy. Any time a change occurs in one member of the family, everybody in the family is affected. Working in individual therapy with an identified patient in a dysfunctional family burdens the individual to become a change agent for the family. This is often too difficult a task for the patient, especially if he or she is a child. Family therapists find it much more efficacious to work at the systems level; in fact, many family therapists refuse to work with individuals. ✻ Family unit - importance!

In our field, we work with families that are under a great deal of stress because they include a person with a communication disorder. These are not necessarily dysfunctional families, only stressed families. Nevertheless, many of the ideas developed by family therapists have profound implications for our field and are beginning to be reflected in our literature.

Egolf, Shames, Johnson, and Kasprisin-Burrell (1972) found that working in the clinic with young persons who stuttered was not sufficient to effect cures, and they recommended that clinicians work with the parent–child dyad. They noted the following:

> If the child adjusts to his environment by stuttering, then the parents must have made an equal adjustment in maintaining stuttering—thus the dyad is in balance (equilibrium). If treatment changes one member of the dyad, the child, by making him fluent, the dyad is forced into disequilibrium. A new equilibrium requires changes in both parent and child. (p. 223)

E. Robertson and Suinn (1968) found a direct correlation between the empathy of family members and the recovery rate of stroke patients. Edgerly (1975) found that a program that provided parent education and tutoring yielded significantly more gains in academic achievement for children with learning disabilities than did a general education program. He concluded that parents must be directly involved in a treatment program for it to be successful. Berry (1987) described techniques and strategies for involving parents in programs for young children using augmentative and alternative communication systems. She concluded that the success of an augmentative communication program is dependent in large part on the attitudes of the family members.

The use of parents dates back to some of our earliest practitioners. Matis (1961) wrote about the need to counsel parents and how it could be done within a single-clinician setting. In language therapy, the recent movement toward pragmatics has brought to the fore the importance of the communicative context, which for children is mainly the family. This means that speech–language pathologists (SLPs) need to involve themselves with the family. In a comprehensive article on family and language intervention, Lund (1986) commented:

> In the family context the child learns a style of relating as well as vocabulary and grammar that will be carried into all subsequent communication situations. We want to highlight and learn from those aspects of the family's interaction that promote effective communication and work with the family to decrease those aspects that seem to impede communication. (p. 417)

Superior and Leichook (1986) argued cogently for involving the parents in a school-based language intervention program. They believed that increased knowledge on the part of the parents about the language disorder would lead to more acceptance and greater sensitivity concerning the restrictions that their children might encounter. They also felt that including the parents would lead to greater carryover into the home environment and to preventive education. If the parents could learn to become strong language models who would facilitate growth in the child's language, the development of further disorders could be prevented. The authors developed a parent-consultation model to be implemented in a public school setting. Girolametta, Greenberg, and Manolson (1986) described a parent program for developing parents' dialogue skills with their children. Andrews (1986), a trained family therapist who works in conjunction with a speech–language pathologist, described techniques for treating language disorders within a family-based approach.

The literature contains little information about the families of adults with catastrophic illness, and few programs seem to be available. After a careful review of the literature on families of persons with aphasia, Emerson (1980) concluded that "involving the family in rehabilitation is more often stressed in theory than actually practiced" (p. 23). He provided a group experience for the spouses of patients with aphasia and found that after group therapy, the spouses displayed gains in self-esteem and were less depressed than were those in a control group that had had no therapy. Within the spouse group, opportunity was provided for the exploration and confirmation of feelings. In conjunction with a speech–language pathologist, Bardach (1969) conducted group sessions with wives of patients with aphasia. She found that these group sessions were immensely helpful and she, like almost everyone who has written in the field, lamented the lack of support programs for families. M. Webster (1982), an adult who suffered a cerebrovascular accident, stated that "had someone been able to counsel with my family about what to expect from me, their lives would have been much easier" (p. 235).

Malone (1969) interviewed the families of 20 adults with aphasia. He found that the aphasia created severe stress for the family, which in turn aggravated the condition of the patient. Probably the most pervasive change noted was role reversal—Wives who had been taken care of by their husbands were suddenly themselves caretakers; husbands who had never assumed any domestic responsibility were now required to do housework in addition to continuing as the breadwinners; children were now required to take care of parents. Families were further stressed by financial problems, health problems, and severe alterations to their social lives. Not surprisingly, these changes generated feelings of guilt and anger. The guilt arose from a feeling that the aphasia was a punishment for a wrong done; the anger was caused by the loss of control.

Kommers and Sullivan (1979) gathered questionnaire data from the wives of men who had had laryngectomies. They found problems in health, communication, finances, and occupation. More than 50% of the younger wives reported marital changes after the laryngectomy. This study did not provide any interview material, but I think it safe to assume that many of the same difficulties that affected the families of the person with aphasia would be shown to affect the families of the men with the laryngectomies.

Alpiner (1978) also found little in the literature about the families of adults with acquired hearing loss. He recommended that the audiologist see the family initially without the member with the hearing impairment to help them understand the hearing loss. He then suggested that if possible, family members should attend therapy sessions.

Fleming (1972) proposed what is essentially a family counseling approach with adults who were hard of hearing. After a comprehensive audiologic workup, the person with the hearing impairment was urged to attend group sessions accompanied by a family member. At these sessions, the families worked out strategies for coping with the hearing impairment, and they also had an opportunity to vent and share their feelings. For example, in one session I attended, a wife was complaining bitterly about being a "hearing-ear dog" for her husband; she was tired of having to answer the phone, explain the punch lines of jokes, and translate television programs. She received confirmation of her feelings from the other spouses in the group, and—with the help of the audiologist who was present—she and her husband were able to devise some techniques to increase his adaptation to the hearing loss. This couple was able to obtain amplifiers for the phone and the television; they also were able to work out some living strategies that would minimize his dependency. In addition, the cathartic experience within the group setting enabled the couple to work constructively on the problem once the interfering feelings had been discharged.

I think the field of communication disorders is gradually coming to realize the efficacy of working at the family level. Federal legislation such as the Education of the Handicapped Act Amendments of 1986 (P.L. 99-457) mandates our involvement at the family level. I think also that as we mature as a profession and throw off our technician shackles, we are recognizing the need to work at a family level. In order to do this successfully, we need to understand how the family system functions and the various roles that significant family members play.

Family Members

Spouses

All marriages involve a contract (Sager, 1978), which is a set of expectations and promises that may or may not be shared with the spouse. More often than not, the contract is implied. There are three levels of contracts: (a) conscious and verbalized, (b) conscious and not verbalized, and (c) unconscious. The marital partners enter their relationship with separate contractual expectations and then work toward developing a joint marital contract. The early conflicts that couples have are usually part of a healthy process of forging this contract.

A major source of marital conflict occurs when there is contractual disappointment. Despite the marriage vow "in sickness and in health," one never really expects or is prepared to deal with severe long-term disability in a spouse. Each marriage partner is usually psychologically protected against thinking about or planning for spousal disability by the myth of invulnerability that we all use to assuage our anxiety over dealing with existential issues. Each spouse has a dream of what marriage and life will be like—a dream that does not include a spousal disability. When a marriage partner becomes disabled by, for example, a stroke or severe hearing loss, the contract is violated. The nondisabled spouse usually is enormously angry and feels somehow cheated. He or she is grief stricken at the loss of the dream and usually feels guilty, believing that he or she did something to cause the disability. The spouse recognizes his or her own vulnerability and is very frightened and anxious about the future. Above all else, the spouse will feel an overwhelming loneliness due to the loss of a marital partner with whom he or she had planned to share his or her life. One man in a disability group I was facilitating lamented, "I have lost my best friend."

Many individuals have nobody with whom to share the burden of caring for the spouse who is disabled. At the time of diagnosis or early signs of the disease, the crisis usually pulls a family together. Short-term difficulties cause people in the family to set aside their personal agendas and rise above individual problems in order to help one another; the immediate crisis has a way of bringing out the best in most people. Later, when family members realize the person has a permanent disability and the problem will be long-term, anger and resentments emerge, and the disappointments become a divisive factor in many families. The well spouse is usually left "holding the bag." This loneliness is acute. Many marriages founder because of the disability of a spouse (or the illness in a child), but many others are strengthened by the crisis.

The marital subsystem within the family is generally delicately balanced and is always seeking equilibrium. In addition to being a contract, a marriage is also a balancing act; partners generally marry someone who has qualities that they admire and feel are lacking in themselves. For example, people with a cognitive bent are usually attracted to mates who deal with the world from an intuitive, feeling stance. This is what sociologists call "marrying complementary," and within the family unit, very often there is a congruence of characteristics that is absent in any one member of the marital pair. If one person is outgoing, the other is usually inhibited; if one is a talker, the other is a listener; and so forth. This is useful to the family during times of crisis; when one spouse is emotionally and cognitively devastated, the other is able to keep the family afloat by dealing with all the information that needs to be processed. The equilibrium is maintained almost unconsciously. I remember a wife complaining that her husband never seemed to grieve over their child's deafness; he was always cheering her up because she was often a "basket case." It wasn't until a year later that he suddenly broke down and cried. It was no accident that his letting go coincided with his wife's feeling good about her ability to cope; this now gave him permission to grieve. Unfortunately, in some families, one adult will get locked into the "up" role and never have space or permission to grieve. When partners are locked into their emotional and physical roles, there invariably is a great deal of marital stress because there is a restriction on each individual's ability to grow.

If one person in a couple has a chronic illness, the complementary and supportive nature of the relationship is lost. The well partner has to go it alone in a caretaker role, and the loneliness can beome extreme. These people are living in chronic grief, constantly mourning for the life before the illness and having to accept the life with the illness. It is in essence an ongoing funeral without any of the societal and ritualistic supports we give to the newly bereaved. In her memoir of living with a husband with a severe disability, Cohen (1996) wrote that she felt like a "separate species," totally alienated from her environment. The only place she felt understood and emotionally supported was within a caregiver support group. One husband of a woman with a severe disability had this to say: "Her life is elemental and focused; getting through the affairs of daily living are about all she can accomplish. She is not striving for much of anything else other than survival and who can help her manage her next bowel movement. There is not much left over to be a wife."

The loneliness is accompanied by immense anger, which is a result of the violation of a life expectation, a loss of control, and fear. The fear is primal and a result of a threat to the basic security of the person. This is a mid-brain response not under the immediate control of the cortex. For example, I would get furious whenever my wife dropped anything, which she was very inclined to do. My anger was related to the fear that she would shortly need to be fed, which would subtantially increase my caregiving burden. I can see this dynamic when I can step back from it; at the time, I am to close to it to do anything about it.

Clinicians working with persons who are chronically ill and their families must learn to deal with the anger and respond to the underlying fear, which is not an easy thing to do but one that can be very fruitful for the family.

Predominant Fears of Nondisabled Spouses or Partners

1. *Progression of the Disease.* Progression is always a threat that overhangs the family as they recognize their vulnerability. It is a challenge to the current

family homeostasis and will require family members to learn new skills and make changes in how they live. It is also a further move down the disability path that assaults the bubble of denial in which most families with chronic illness live.

2. *Health of the Caregiver.* Most persons are living within a nuclear family system. For most caregivers, extended family is not available. As a result, the caregiving burden falls on one or two members. This means the family has no fail-safe margin if the caregiver becomes ill. The stress of caregiving is enormous, and the family is at constant risk. One of the first topics that emerges in caregiver groups is "Who can take over if I am sick?" All families with a disability live in constant terror concerning the caregiver's health.

3. *Vulnerability of the Children.* Many of the autoimmune diseases are inheritable, which puts the children more at risk for developing one of these diseases. This is a fear that seldom is discussed by the marital pair. I remember that in one support group, a wife of a man with multiple sclerosis announced that her daughter had just been diagnosed with the disease. It wiped everyone out emotionally, including me. It is probably equated with the greatest fear any parent has—the death of a child.

4. *Economic Devastation.* Our society is doing a poor job of supporting families with chronic illness. The expense can be enormous and catastrophic. In order for a family to receive government help for nursing home care, they must qualify for Medicaid, which means they must essentially be impoverished. To keep a person who is chronically ill at home often requires support personnel, including speech–language pathologists, for which there is limited governmental and insurance help despite the fact that this option is often less expensive than placement in a nursing home. The spectre of economic devastation hangs over many families where there is a chronic illness and frequently leads to a decision by family members to try to care for the patient on their own, often with inadequate skills or resources. This is seldom in the patient's best interest, and many families are at risk because the caretakers become overwhelmed or incapacitated.

5. *Adequacy.* All caregivers wonder whether or not they will be able to stay the course. Many chronic illnesses require the caregiver to learn new skills and to constantly adjust emotionally to a new reality. This stresses the family system, and the primary caregiver in particular, and at times is overwhelming. Divorce rates in families with chronic illness are high, and instances of caregiver illness are also numerous. My wife often wondered, as did I, whether or not we would be adequate enough to bear the burden of this disease with grace and dignity.

6. *Is This a Life Sentence?* This question is pondered almost daily by both the person with the chronic illness and his or her family. Many, if not all, of

these diseases are life sentences—there is no cure, no getting better. In one support group, a husband of a wife with Parkinson's disease said, "A friend called me the other day to tell me that his wife has terminal cancer. I commiserated with him, but when I hung up the phone I thought how lucky he was." We all understood instantly what he meant. At least with the terminal illness, awful as it may be, there is a time limitation and the caregiver can plan for a noncaregiving future. My wife had multiple sclerosis for 30 years, and she could have easily gone another 20 years, albeit severely disabled. In moments of despair, I had been heard to mutter, "By the time I finish caregiving, I will need it."

The biggest fear that the identified patient has is abandonment. This is a function of dependency, and the greater the disability and the fewer the number of available caregivers, the greater the fear.

I again want to remind the reader that these fears are present in almost all families where there is a chronic illness, and they will manifest themselves as anger. Productive counseling can be best accomplished by responding to the fear and not the anger. Helping the person identify the fear often leads to productive behavior. For example, awareness of economic fear can lead to gathering insurance and financial trust information and eventually to behavior that reduces the fear and thus the anger.

In a comprehensive article on couples with a neurological disability, Ventimiglia (1986) listed factors that would lead to the preservation of the marital relationship; among them were the following:

1. *If the disability is mild and remains stable.* Change is hard to deal with because it stresses the system to accommodate the new reality, raising anew feelings of inadequacy. When there is stability, the system accommodates it, and this becomes "normal." There were so many things that I had to do for my wife that I didn't think about them until I was on a trip and realized I didn't have to take care of anyone else but myself. It was so easy. I could live comfortably in my abnormal "normal" until I had to adjust to a new reality, and then the grief and fear began anew. When the disorder is mild, it is easy to deny. We had to make very few changes in our lifestyle for the first 10 years after the initial diagnosis. The fear was always there but was generally dormant. It wasn't until the disease progressed to the point of us having to make significant accommodations in our lifestyle that stress began to emerge in our marital relationship.

2. *If there is an abundance of resources.* As mentioned previously, caring for persons with chronical illness requires many resources, both economic and social. To accommodate increasing physical disability, my wife and I had to extensively modify our home. We added a lift in the house and built a bedroom and "handicapped" bath. I had to use some of my early retirement pay to accom-

plish this. We also had to hire home-health aides and respite workers so I could have some relief. Fortunately, we had the resources, but many families do not.

Social resource are as important as financial ones. It is easy for the family to spiral down into lonely misery. Many of the activities that the couple formerly did with other couples are now denied to them, and friends slowly drop away as activities become limited. This usually occurs gradually, until the well spouse wakes up one day and realizes just how lonely and limited he or she is. Divorces are made of such revelations.

3. *If the marital contract is renegotiated.* As mentioned before, at their heart, all marriages are contractual arrangements. In a marriage were there is a person with a disability, expectations must be made explicit and renegotiated. Nothing destroys relationships more than the anger that results from unmet implicit expectations. Because many chronic illnesses have a progressive characteristic, the contract must be constantly renegotiated. My wife and I were constantly searching for ways that she could contribute to our family functioning. In order to succeed, couples often must be taught the skill of communicating their wants and needs to each other.

4. *If tolerable substitions are made for lost activities.* Many chronic illnesses place physical limitations on activities the couple formerly enjoyed together. This is equally true if the partner with a disability has a cognitive deficit or a communication disorder. My wife and I were very active, running 10-K races and hiking. These activities became things of the past. Instead we read to each other, listened to the radio, and watched old movies on television. Not the same, but good nonetheless.

5. *If some philosophical sense is made of the life situation.* Couples must find an answer to the "Why us?" question. Not to do so dooms them to living in anger and bitterness, which they invariably take out on each other. Reframing is an incredibly valuable tool for the clinician and the couple to use if the couple is receptive. I prefer to think of these disorders as the powerful teachers that they are. Another reframing that I find helpful is the idea that although life may have dealt me a lousy "hand," it is still my task to play well the "cards" I have been dealt.

6. *If the well spouse is prone to nurturance.* Men are more likely to leave a spouse with a disability than are women. I think women are generally acculturated into a nuturing role and it is not as much of a role reversal for a woman to become a caretaker for her partner. For men it is often a greater leap. I have seen families in which the man is inclined towards nurturance; these families usually do well. Another reason a woman may be more inclined to "hang in there" is economic. Many older women cannot survive financially on their own because they do not have the skills to earn a living and therefore feel forced to stay in a desperate situation.

7. *If the couple receive help.* I believe that a support group can become a primary vehicle for healing. It is often the only place the nondisabled marriage partner gets validation of his or her feelings and also receives information on coping strategies. This is equally true for the partner with the disability. I have found that it is best to put members of a couple into separate groups. Couples' groups are very difficult to manage because the nondisabled individual is often inhibited by the presence of his or her spouse. When caregivers start to reveal how hard it is for them, the partner with the disability often feels threatened and gets defensive. It becomes hard for the partners to hear each other. I think couples' work is best accomplished after each partner has had an opportunity to vent within his or her own support group. A couples' group can then become productive.

Staying within a disability marriage and flourishing is very difficult and cannot be done successfully without a lot of professional and nonprofessional help. Many of these marriages end in divorce or become hollow shells. Ventimiglia (1986) commented that in many cases, "Divorce becomes a matter of survival, not the pursuit of happiness" (p. 125). In my experience of working with groups of healthy spouses of persons who have a chronical illness I have found that the couples who grow and prosper through the adversity of the disability are the older, longer-married individuals whose companionship has been tested over time. The other type of partnership that succeeds is the newly married couple where the well person entered the marriage knowing about the disability and openly and honestly made his or her choice. No matter how well prepared people may think they are for a disability marriage, they really cannot know how they will react until they live it. The pain ultimately wears down a well spouse. Caring for someone on a short-term basis or only in a peripheral capacity is relatively easy; one can be loving and giving if he or she can plan to return to a normal life in a short while.

The persons most at risk are individuals who have been married for only a few years and have not been subjected to enough external stress to strengthen them, or those who have not yet established openness in their marital communication. These marriages are much more likely to crumble under the added weight of a disability.

Having a spouse with a chronic disability does not necessarily lead to divorce or estrangement. The disability causes marital stress by altering the marriage contract and violating expectations, thus exposing weaknesses that might otherwise have been "papered over." With some marriages, the exposed cracks are so deep that the foundation crumbles. In other marriages, the stress caused by the disability is an occasion for working and strengthening the marital bond and cementing the cracks so that a stronger foundation can be put in place.

The professional in communication disorders needs to direct considerable clinical attention to the nondisabled spouse. This is time well spent and can have an enormous long-term impact on the client. By supporting and educating the spouse, the professional can help create a home that is facilitative for the client. Unfortunately, this does not happen often enough. In a spousal group I was facilitating, one wife said, "I have had multiple sclerosis for 17 years, only nobody knows it." Another spouse said, "In this concert I am always playing second violin." Programmatically, we need to look at these "second fiddles."

We need to redirect our professional energies toward making the well spouse our first priority; if we take good care of him or her (as with the parents), the patient will usually do well. We need to include the spouse in all diagnostic workups as well as in therapy with the client. Rollins (1988) described completely the reactions of spouses of person with aphasia and the implications for counseling; he recommended actively involving the spouse in therapy and diagnosis. Some spouses are so locked in denial and anger that it seems we cannot reach them. We need to listen to and support them as we work to enhance their self-esteem. They may then give up denial; as we listen and avoid judgment, they may have a chance to vent their anger.

Above all else, we must provide a support group in which some of that crushing loneliness can be abated. Having worked intensively with spousal groups for the past several years, I have become ever more certain of the value of support groups in providing a healing environment.

In the early sessions of a well spouse group, there is an immense sense of relief and a rush of long pent-up emotions that emerges like a dam bursting: It is almost palpable. Finally, other people understand what the well spouses are going through, and they can be accepted as they talk about their problems without feeling guilty or whining. After the first few sessions, which are mainly cathartic, group members usually begins sharing information as they move from an emotion-centered focus to a problem-centered one. Spouses leave feeling supported; they have established a network of friends that can relieve the crushing loneliness of living with a person who has a chronic illness.

Parents

According to Minuchin (1974), modern parenting is essentially an impossible task. He stated, and I agree wholeheartedly, that "parenting is an extremely difficult task that no one performs to his entire satisfaction and no one goes through the process unscathed" (p. 83). There is always conflict. Parents cannot protect and guide a child without at times being controlling and restrictive.

On the other hand, children cannot grow without testing the limits imposed by their parents and seeming rejecting and hostile. Parents often are in conflict not only with their children but also with themselves as to whether they are fulfilling their nurturing function or their controlling–guiding function. The chronic dilemma of all parents is determining in a given situation how much control they should maintain and how much freedom they should give to their children. The parents' job is to gradually cede control to the child, but the timing of the release of control is very difficult to determine. If parents cede control too quickly, the child will have negative experiences that can lead to feelings of incompetency. If the parents hold on too long, the child will receive the message that he or she is not competent to deal with the world. Both premature and delayed release of control generally have the same result: a fearful, low-risk child. There is a relatively small margin of control with which the responsible parent has to work; a disability in the child limits the margins even further.

According to Satir (1967), "The parents are the axis around which all other family relationships are formed. The mates are the architects of the family" (p. 63). The marital relationship affects parenting: When parents are close and supportive of each other, they are better able to fulfill their parental responsibilities. When parents are not emotionally close, very often the child gets "triangulated" into the marriage. Triangulation often occurs when the child is born with a disability, and as discussed earlier, the child may develop psychosomatic symptoms in order to salvage the marriage.

According to Mendelsohn and Rozek (1983), the "intrinsic characteristics of the deafness and the caretaking process lend themselves to the child being easily triangulated into the anxious or conflictual areas in the family's life. The disability puts the child into focus more easily because of the need for more attention and care" (p. 39). Pedersen (1976) studied families with a child with a disability and found that when there was a husband who was emotionally distant, the wife was also. A mother's ability to parent well is a function in large part of the satisfaction she obtains in her marriage. Gallagher, Cross, and Scharfman (1981) identified the characteristics of parents who were judged by professionals to have made a successful adjustment to the birth of a child with a disability. The data suggested that the major sources of strength were the personal qualities of the parents and the quality of the husband–wife relationship.

The triangle consisting of the parents and the child is most apparent in preschool programs, where it is not uncommon to find a father who is emotionally distant. Programs usually try to strengthen the father–child bond by seducing the father into involvement with the program. For example, a fairly recent conference of educators of individuals with hearing impairments devoted an entire session to involving fathers in home intervention (Ski Hi, 1985). Among the suggestions developed were to establish rapport with the father early, take time to write or leave notes for him, call him at work, give him assignments, and always reinforce him for his work with the child. I think these strategies will work nicely in families in which the father is timid about involving himself with his child. This is especially true for first-time fathers of very young children. It must be kept in mind that system theory would predict that when the father–child relationship is altered, the mother–child relationship and the husband–wife relationship will be altered as well. One leg of the triangle cannot change without affecting the other legs.

Very often, however, the attempts to attract the father fail completely or succeed only momentarily before the father resumes his distant behavior. Invariably, the professional starts searching for another gimmick to attract the father or enters into a subtle coalition with the mother that only further excludes and alienates the father. This is always a mistake.

We professionals can affect the father–child relationship by working with the mother–child dyad or the husband–wife relationship. In families with fathers who are distant, the mothers frequently are very closely bonded to their children, sometimes to the point that they do not want the father present at all, despite their protestations to the contrary. Many of these mothers have unresolved feelings of guilt, and they feel that repairing the "damage" is their responsibility. For many mothers, the children with a disability also become the means for realizing their self-worth; they discover the joy of working with their children and gain confidence in their ability to do the job well. In essence, the children give direction and meaning to their lives; consequently, they do not want the fathers to "mess up" their work. Frequently in these situations, a father is insecure and lacks competence in doing what needs to be done, and the mother would rather do it herself. She either consciously or unconsciously excludes or intimidates him.

The presence of a child with a disability often triggers a spiral into marital discord. When the mother becomes overinvolved with the child, little energy is left for the marriage. When the father is getting little satisfaction within the marriage, he will seek involvement somewhere else—usually work. As he becomes more involved in work, she becomes more involved in parenting, which leaves him to become further involved in work, and so it goes until there is little or no energy left for the marriage.

Some wives need to have a club to wield over their husbands. The father's physical and emotional distance from the child with a disability often becomes that weapon. The mother frequently gets emotional support from other family members and sometimes from professionals for her feelings about the "bad" father because she is "doing it" alone. It is always poor case management for the speech–language pathologist or audiologist to enter into an alliance with the mother against the father. If we examined the marriage closely, we would invariably find a great deal of conflict; the fight over the child is usually only one of many long-simmering disputes.

Another thing to bear in mind is that some families can be quite successful with a father who is clinically distant. Because families work in many different ways, professionals need to respect the individual family's coping strategy as long as the family remains functional. A coping strategy that requires an over-involved mother may be necessary if the family is to turn out a successfully functioning child who has a disability. This solution will work if the mother feels that she is supported and that her burden is shared with the family; the father who assumes some of the mother's chores at home while she is at the child's school is emotionally supportive of her and can be a very effective father who never appears at the clinic. There may be no need for him to enter the clinic or be involved directly with his child's therapy. Sometimes there is much truth in the statement that the best thing a father can do for his children is to love his wife.

Female professionals who are at a different stage of social consciousness than the children's mothers often judge a family as deficient if it is run with traditional gender-role stereotypes. These families can be, and very often are, quite successful and functional as long as everyone is content with his or her role. The family must always be accepted for what it is rather than for what the professional feels it should be. We must always be sensitive to multicultural differences among families and never impose our values on the families with whom we are working.

In the Emerson College program, we make no special efforts to coax fathers to attend, although they are always very welcome. We offer evening meetings, or we have a Saturday nursery each semester to accommodate working parents. These are offered only if the parents request them. I have worked with many families in the program without ever meeting the fathers or having only limited contact with them. Many single-parent families are also successful in the program.

The emotions involved in having a child with a disability are intense. Featherstone (1980) noted that a child's disability strains the marriage by evoking such strong emotions in both parents that it becomes "a fertile source of conflict and disrupts the organization of the family. On a long-term basis the disabled child is always a symbol of a shared failure" (p. 172). Gath (1977) studied 30 families with a child with down syndrome for 5 years after the birth of the child, as well as a carefully controlled group of 30 families with nondisabled children. At the end of the 5-year period she found that 9 of the families with the child with down syndrome experienced severe marital discord, whereas none of the control families reported this kind of difficulty.

Anger is probably the emotion that is potentially most destructive to the marriage. The parents usually have no satisfactory outlet for anger. Many do not even recognize their anger; others repress it, and it emerges as depression. In families where the expression of anger is not sanctioned, anger is often displaced; for example, the parents may argue about the quality of the cooking or the whiteness of the laundry. In the early stages of diagnosis and therapy, the parents' fights are seldom over what actually angers them. The loss of control and the impotence they feel in the face of their child's disability fuel many a fight. Much of the anger is also displaced onto the professionals.

Guilt is also potentially destructive to a marriage if it is not recognized and dealt with effectively. Guilt is usually felt by both parents, although mothers—because they carried the child during pregnancy—seem to carry a heavier load. Because guilt is such an uncomfortable feeling, the parents try to push it off on each other. They search through their family trees to find some defective relative, preferably on the other partner's side. In combination with rage, guilt can be a formidably divisive force. The anger and blame that parents feel has split up many a marriage.

With guilt often comes the "super-dedicated" parent who is committed to "making it up" to the child with a disability, usually at the expense of the rest of the family. Less attention is paid to the husband–wife relationship and to the nondisabled siblings. The parent often ignores his or her own needs and becomes undimensional, almost monomaniacal. The child's disability becomes the dominating force in the family, to the exclusion and resentment of everyone else. If allowed to, the child with a disability can consume an inordinate amount of energy and radically alter the family structure.

In most families, the parents do not synchronize their feelings or are unwilling to share their feelings because they feel they would be imposing on the other. For example, a mother in a parent group spoke about not wanting to tell her husband her fears and anxieties because that just "sets him off." She kept stating, "We aren't very good for each other because we pull each other down." It is also difficult to deal with one parent who is heavily in denial while the other is obviously deeply distressed. Each parent feels that he or she lacks support from the other, and each feels that his or her spouse does not understand what is occurring.

Frequently a spouse finds it difficult to listen and respond to their partner's pain. This seems especially true of husbands. Men frequently assign themselves the role of family protector, and when a member of their family is in pain about which they can do nothing, they feel responsible. This emotion often triggers a denial reaction. Many men refuse to talk about feelings because to do so undermines their own denial mechanism. They then try to distract their wives from the pain in order to make the wives feel better, usually with disastrous results.

(In actuality, they are trying to make themselves feel better, and this needs to be pointed out.) The inability or unwillingness of parents to talk about their feelings can be very divisive. The professional needs to help the parents resolve the issue of managing each other's grief. He or she needs to be a person with whom parents can talk and cry without having their feelings invalidated. It is often desirable to bring both parents together to discuss the dynamics of their relationship as it is affected by grief, and it is often necessary to try to release the husband from the protector role in order to allow him to grieve and to leave space in the relationship for the wife's grief.

Yalom (1989) said the following about working with grieving parents:

> Therapy has much to offer grieving parents. Couples' treatment may illuminate the source of marital tension and help each partner to recognize and respect the other's mode of grief. Individual therapy may help to alter dysfunctional mourning. Wary though I am always of generalizations, in this instance male–female stereotypes also hold true. Many women need to move past the repetitive expression of their loss and to plunge back into engagement with the living, with projects, with all the things that may supply meaning for their own lives. Men usually must be taught to experience and share (rather than to suppress and evade) their sadness. (p. 142)

Many changes in the family structure occur when a child with a disability is introduced. The husband–wife relationship is altered radically, wives may have to postpone their careers even further, and economic hardships can occur. Plans are formulated based on the availability of schooling, and difficult family choices often have to be made. Families often need a place to talk about these changes and their stresses. In many programs, parent education becomes, in fact, mother education. Very often the mother, by virtue of being actively involved in the educational program, possesses more information and is in a better position to make decisions regarding the child's welfare than is the father. In some families that have a very set gender-role orientation, the changing role of the wife can be a threat to marital stability. Over the 35-year history of the Emerson College program, we have seen several marriages founder. I am not sure that the number of failed marriages in this population is any greater than in the general population as a whole, which is alarming, but clearly the child with a disability does add more stress to the marriage. I do not consider divorce a failure. Very often it is a solution, albeit a painful one, to a difficult situation. I think children are better off in a family in which the parents divorce than in a family in which there is no communication or love between the parents. The divorce also sometimes leads to the spouse who keeps the child finding the external support that he or she didn't have while married.

In the Emerson College program, families are the central element. In addition to attending the support group once a week, parents are required to participate with their child in the nursery at least one morning a week. The nursery is staffed by an early childhood professional instead of a teacher of the deaf. (The Emerson College program is for children with hearing impairments, but the discerning reader can see that this format is appropriate for children with other disabilities as well.) I think it is important that we pay attention to the human needs first and then to the special needs of the deafness. To this end, we always try to include in the nursery a hearing child, not to stimulate language so much as to remind us all of the developmental issues of a 2-year-old. One chronic problem that parents have is trying to distinguish between the behavior that is due to the hearing loss and the behavior that is due to developmental issues. One fantasy that parents often have is, "If I could just speak to my child, all of the problems would clear up." They realize this is a fantasy when they watch staff members try to deal with the hearing child. The mother of the hearing child also participates in the parent group, and the mothers of the children with the hearing impairment usually realize that this mother is having as many management problems as they are. (Probably the deafest creature on the face of the earth is a 2-year-old, with or without a hearing loss.)

Usually eight children between the ages of 18 months and 3 years are in the nursery with the nursery school teacher and several graduate students from a speech-pathology program. The nursery is equipped with a large one-way mirror through which parents observe their children. The children have individual speech–language therapy each day in adjoining therapy rooms, also equipped with one-way mirrors for parental observation. As the program progresses (we operate on an academic calendar from September to May), the parents begin to take over the program. Instead of watching, they take turns working with the children in the nursery and in therapy while staff members watch. By springtime, it is often hard to tell through casual observation who are the staff members and who are the parents. At all points we seek to empower the parents.

Over the years, our definition of "parent" has evolved because so many mothers work now, and the traditional family where the mother stays home and the father works is rare. We will enroll any family as long as a primary caregiver is present. We have worked on occasion with aunts, grandparents, and babysitters. We will not enroll any child without an accompanying caregiver. We feel it is presumptuous to think that by working 5 or 6 hours a week with only the child, we can effect massive changes; however, by spending that time with the adults, we can affect the child all the time by helping to change the home environment. It is much more efficacious to work this way than to work solely with the child.

Fathers seldom receive or solicit emotional support; almost all support seems to be directed toward the mothers. Many fathers *do* need to be heard and to be able to talk about their feelings—a fact they may not even realize. Programs need to provide opportunities for the fathers to participate without stressing the marital contract. Fathers can be invited, and if they do not attend, that needs to be accepted as well.

Crowley, Keane, and Needham (1982) held a series of bimonthly evening meetings with fathers of children enrolled in a school for the deaf. During the first year, they offered a rather structured, content-based program; later they moved into an unstructured group discussion that encouraged more self-disclosure and feelings. Both fathers and staff members concluded that the program was very successful. I suspect that the more structured, content-based program was a good entry point for the fathers. Most men seem to find it difficult to talk about feelings, and if some trust and cohesion can be developed in the group while dealing with structured content, it may be easier for the men to move subsequently into affect areas.

In the Emerson College program, we have held nursery on a Saturday morning at least once each semester so that fathers could attend. We have had evening group meetings with fathers only, and we have had husband-and-wife groups. In the latter groups, it was difficult to get much openness, as each parent did not want to reveal very much for fear of angering the other. One semester we held a group in which half the men and half the women attended, but they were not spouses of each other. We held a second meeting with the other halves; these groups were a great deal more open, and there was a strong confidentiality norm.

We have also experimented with intensive weekend experiences that did not include the children. Staff members and parents spend 2 days together in a resort setting where time is set aside for reflection and recreation as well as for group meetings. Within this setting, I have used a "fishbowl design" where half of the group sits in the center and the other half is silent and on the periphery. The fathers, for example, may talk about how they are affected by their children's deafness while the mothers listen, then the mothers talk while the fathers listen. At the end of the session, everybody processes the experience; I always try to conclude an intense husband–wife encounter, with the couples going off to a corner and taking turns telling each other what they appreciate about the other person. Other sessions are devoted to large-group discussions. The fishbowl, in conjunction with the intensive weekend experience, has given us very cohesive parent groups. There has been greater father participation and involvement in all aspects of the program when we have been able to use the intensive weekend; unfortunately, for the past several years, costs have precluded our using this strategy. I have also worked with programs for deaf children that include a learning vacation for the families. I find that there is the same intensity of experience in these groups as there are in the clinic-based programs, and they are among the most satisfying that I do, albeit on a very short-term basis.

My experience has suggested that although the presence of a child with a disability in the family creates stress, there are also significant positives for many families. For example, the stress can be an occasion for growth. Kazak and Marvin (1984) found that in 56 families in which a child had spina bifida, a significant portion of the parents reported that their marriage was strengthened as a result. A mother of a 5-year-old child who was deaf told me,

> I really grew to appreciate my husband these last few years. He has really risen to the occasion. He has gone with me to all important meetings, and he takes over a great deal of the day-to-day responsibility from me. I never knew he cared so deeply for me and my child until this happened.

The professional who works sensitively with the family members when there is a child with a disability can help them achieve a positive outcome from the experience. I think a major key to working with the parents is to give them permission to take care of themselves first. A valuable metaphor for me has been the instructions I receive from the flight attendant whenever I fly. I am told that if an oxygen mask should be needed and I am traveling with a child, I should put a mask on my face first and then take care of the child. This makes powerful sense to me because in order to give, I have to be getting from someplace, and if I go under, there is nobody to take care of the child. If I am to take good care of somebody else, I have to start by taking good care of myself. Parents often don't see this simple truth; they tend to give and give until they are burnt out and resentful. If they do something for themselves, they usually feel guilty. One thing I have learned in the past 40 years of doing clinical work is that happy parents turn out well-functioning children. If they can take some time for themselves and for their marriages, they will be better parents. The counseling program needs to provide an avenue for the parents to find their happiness. Each time I work with a parent group, I am struck anew by how much growth and joy can emerge from so much pain and suffering.

The Children of Disability

The need to view one's parents as strong, intelligent, and very competent is a childhood illusion that is difficult to alter at any age, It is hard to know when childhood ends; we have no real markers. My brother has commented that the time he was most frightened while growing up was when he talked about a family problem and our parents actually listened to him.

Adolescents are normally granted a moratorium or postponement period during which the identity of childhood gradually merges with that of adulthood. Eventually the adolescent must give up this moratorium to assume adult responsibility. Adolescence is a cultural and social event. The biology is clear: One moment you are a child, and the next minute you are capable of having children. Adolescence is a luxury that society can afford only when it is affluent. In marginal societies, the adolescent joins the workforce in order to contribute to the society as soon as possible, and in poor families in an affluent society, the adolescent is often called on to assume adult responsibilities sooner than his or her better-off counterparts. For example, my father, the son of immigrant parents, left school after the eighth grade to join the workforce and become an important financial contributor to the family. He never had an adolescence and could not cope very well with mine (I don't know many parents who can); we had a stormy relationship until shortly before his death.

Probably the best indication of when someone has arrived at adulthood is the willingness to see one's parents as fellow adults struggling with the very human problems of making the most of their lives. There is a predictable life crisis of adulthood that occurs when we realize that we are more capable than our parents. This is not the adolescent experience that Mark Twain described when he quipped, "When I was 15, I thought my father was the stupidest person alive. At 19, I was surprised at how much he had learned in 4 short years."

There does come a time for all of us, usually in our adulthood, when we realize that we really do know more than our parents. A role reversal occurs, and we begin to parent our parents. This realization usually leaves us feeling frightened and alone because we often experience for the first time our existential aloneness and recognize that there is nobody left to protect us. For most of us, the realization that we must care for our parents usually occurs over time, fueled by many small incidents that reflect our parents' increasing incompetence.

For adolescent children of a parent with a disability, the moratorium phase is shortened or sometimes is even nonexistent as they become "parentified" and are forced to assume adult responsibilities much sooner than their peers. For these children, the normal crisis of adulthood is accelerated. They have to deal with parental incompetence at a much earlier age than they might be ready for developmentally. This can be quite frightening to self-absorbed adolescents, who ordinarily see parents as unwanted intrusions on their autonomy, or merely as providers for their sustenance, but rarely as people. To have to suddenly look at your father as a person who is hurting and fearful and who may now be dependent on you is quite frightening.

There is very little information in the literature specifically on how children of disability fare. In a careful review of the literature on children of adults with a disability, Roy (1990) concluded, "How much attention should the clinician pay to the children of chronically ill parents? Common sense suggests a great deal but research evidence remains equivocal" (p. 120). In my experience of interviewing families and working with them professionally, I have found that the children can either (a) become parentified early and lose their adolescence while becoming responsible young adults, or (b) they act out their fears and perceived lack of attention by getting into trouble. Children can survive and grow under adverse conditions; what they cannot sustain is indifference, and as long as they feel cared for by the parents they will respond and grow. The issue is whether or not the parents have any energy left to deal with their children's problems while they are wrestling with the formidable issues engendered by their own disability.

We do know that children are sensitive barometers of family stress. All writers on the subject agree that life is stressful for the child of a parent with a disability, but the stress can work either way—It can be a maturing factor and produce a very responsible child, or it can lead to neglect and become a springboard for delinquent behavior. It seems to me that the children's success or lack of it is almost always a function of how well the parents are coping with the disease process. When the parents are able to put the disorder in perspective, so that it is no longer dominating their every waking thought and consuming their psychic and physical energy, they can devote time to their children. Until this happens, the children (especially in the early stages of diagnosis) are pretty much on their own. If there was strength in the family to begin with, then the child can survive and even flourish. In weaker family systems, the children—and the family itself—may not be able to survive without considerable scarring.

The effect of parental chronic illness on the adult child who has left the family is also variable, depending in large part on that child's designated role in the family and how close both physically and emotionally that child is to the parent. Some children within the family structure become designated early as caretakers. This role usually devolves onto the oldest girl (see the section on siblings later in this chapter). I have encountered families in which the caretaker was a son, but these have been relatively rare. Most of the research on the adult child of disability has been with Alzheimer's patients. Because the patient is mentally incompetent, researchers are forced to use the family.

Dementia, in particular, is an illness that strikes at the very core of person's humanness, altering the hallmarks of personality and intelligence. The worm of the disease burrows deeply within and destroys a person's substance, leaving only an "empty husk" for others to view. The body remains the same, at least in the early stages, but the mind and personhood, as family members remember it, are gone. There is a psychological death long before the physical death, and there are no rituals to help the family through the mourning. It is a neverending struggle for family members of patients with dementia to try to keep fresh the memory of what used to be while dealing with the present reality, which bears no resemblance in the ways that matter to the person they knew.

One adult child of parent with Alzheimer's disease had this to say in one of my counseling sessions:

> The crazy thing too is that someone has really died 2 years ago, in essence, yet their actual death is still a horrible process. I don't know what you hang on to. You hang on to something. The difficulty is then of getting that memory of the last stages out of your mind. The impressions are so strong. That's not what you want to remember about them. It's hard to bring them back the way they were. It takes a long time when you remember them, not to remember them the way they were at the end. It happens eventually. It takes time.

Children must always struggle with the decision to institutionalize a parent with dementia. Invariably, they have guilt because they feel they are failing in their responsibilities, and for many families, the decision to institutionalize a loved one is an economic decision. At more than $6,000 a month, most families cannot afford for long to keep a family member in a nursing home, so they attempt to care for him or her themselves, usually at horrendous cost to the health and welfare of the rest of the family. The laws are such that families must reduce themselves to a poverty status before they can begin to "afford" a nursing home, and when faced with the twin prospects of poverty or exhaustion, most families opt for exhaustion; the literature is replete with instances where the able-bodied spouse, especially in cases of illness, such as dementia, needed psychiatric care and hospitalization because of the stress caused by the caregiving. Depression and exhaustion are the two most frequent characteristics of the caretakers (Baumgarten et al., 1990). The decision to institutionalize is complex, involving a host of variables, including the amount of family strain, family finances, the support structure of the family, and the health of the primary caretaker (Rabins, 1984).

In any event, the family, especially the adult children, must be able to somehow reconstitute their lives after the death of the parent. Nuland (1994) described the problem very well:

> It often seems as though the families of Alzheimer's patients are sidetracked from the broad sunlit avenues of ongoing life, remaining trapped for years in its own excruciating cul-de-sac. The only rescue comes with the death of a person they love. And even then, the memories and the dreadful toll drag on, and from these the release can only be partial. A life

that has been well lived and a shared sense of happiness and accomplish-ments are ever after seen through the smudged glass of its last few years. For the survivors, the concourse of existence has forever become less bright and less direct. (p. 105)

Perhaps the ultimate act of adulthood is the burying of your parents; for the children of disability, it is not always clear when the death takes place. What is clear is that they are called on to become compassionate, caring adults at an early age, which many of these children seem to accomplish very well.

Grandparents

At this time, there is little published research about grandparents. They often play a very important role in the families that we encounter, but they appear to be a badly underresearched, underused resource to the family and to professionals.

Grandparents are present in every family, whether or not they are actively involved. We always carry our family of origin into our new nuclear family. Our ideas of what constitutes marriage and parenthood stem from our childhood experiences when we observed and assessed our parents' parenting and our par-ents' marriage. We carry that image with us when we start our new family, either by imitating our parents or by determining to be different from them. In either case, we are heavily influenced by them. Only with time and thought do we begin to find our way into marital and parental roles based on our own direct experiences. Some of this change comes about in the initial phases of family for-mation due to the stress of melding the spouses' disparate personal paradigms into a new family paradigm. Our ideas of what is appropriate and normal stem from our experience in our families of origin and reflect the values of our grand-parents.

"Grandparenthood" is the ultimate developmental phase of parenthood. It is being able to parent without having the responsibility. Probably the only peo-ple from whom the child can have unconditional love is the grandparents. Because of their civilizing–instructing function, parents are often in conflict with their children, whereas grandparents generally have more loving and accepting relationships. I always knew that if the police were on my tail, my grandmother would take me in. My parents would also take me in, but they would believe the police. My grandmother would always believe me. A cynic has commented that grandparents and grandchildren are natural allies because they both have the same enemy. It is a rare person who has a bad relationship with his or her grandparent.

Unfortunately, the grandparent seems to be rapidly disappearing as an involved member of the family. Kornhaber and Woodward (1985), who conducted interviews with 300 grandparents and grandchildren, found that only 15% of the families included an actively involved grandparent. The majority (70%) of grandparents were intermittently involved, and 15% were not involved at all. Kornhaber and Woodward felt that a new social contract was in effect that allowed the parents to define the grandparents' role, and this new role was one of diminished grandparent involvement. (I think that the increased affluence that has enabled grandparents to live independently and at a distance from their children also contributes to this diminishing involvement. Extended families used to be a necessity because grandparents could no longer support themselves after retiring; Social Security has changed this.)

Based on their in-depth interviews of the children and the grandparents, Kornhaber and Woodward (1985) found that families benefited from closely connected grandparents. The grandparents functioned as mentors, caretakers, and mediators between the child and the parents; as gender role models; and as family historians. The results of this study suggested no negative effects of grandparent involvement. A different picture might have emerged if the authors had interviewed the parents, because grandparents can and frequently do introduce stress into the home.

There is minimal information in the literature about the grandparents' role in families with a child who has a disability; they are generally the "forgotten" people. For example, a monograph published by the *Volta Review*, "Families and Their Hearing Impaired Children" (Atkins, 1987), has no chapter devoted to grandparents.

Harris, Handiman, and Palmer (1985) used a questionnaire to interview the parents and grandparents of 19 children with autism. They found that the grandparents had a consistently less pessimistic view of the child's limitations than did the parents. They also noted that the grandparents tended to deny the child's disability long after it had been accepted by the parents. Lowe (1989) adapted the Harris et al. questionnaire for grandparents of 39 deaf children. She found similar results, with the grandparents consistently more optimistic and more locked in denial than the parents.

These are the only two empirical studies in the literature concerning grandparents of children with special needs. They both validate my own clinical observations that grandparents generally lag behind the parents in accepting the disability. It is very difficult for the grandparents to deal with the pain of having a grandchild with a disability in conjunction with the pain their own child is experiencing. For the grandparents it is a double hurt, at a time in life when they are least prepared to cope with emotional emergencies. Like most nonprofessionals, the grandparents lack information and knowledge about the child's disorder; consequently, their own children frequently know far more than they do, and a role reversal suddenly occurs. The parents, through their professional contacts and by virtue of living with the problem on a daily basis, generally move through the mourning stages much faster than the grandparents do. When we are hurting, we generally want and need support from our own parents. The parents of the child with a disability, when they seek support from their own parents, often find it is not there. Instead, the grandparents are seek-ing information and support from their own children. The parents are then in a role reversal where they are forced to parent their own parents. They often feel cheated and deeply resentful of this reversal because they themselves want badly to be parented, and the support is not forthcoming.

The parents are also plagued by feelings of guilt vis-à-vis their own parents: One of the "tasks" of children is to produce grandchildren for their parents; it is part of an implicit and sometimes explicit compact that parents and children have. When people have a child with a disability, which causes their parents pain instead of joy, they may feel guilty. Anger very often masks the guilt that the parents feel, and usually a very unhealthy dynamic begins to develop in the parent–grandparent relationship.

Grandparents' feelings parallel closely the parents' responses. They feel grief, anger, anxiety, and guilt in varying proportions. They display their feelings to their children and to professionals in accordance with the cultural values of their family. More often than not, there is no openness about feelings between the grandparents and the parents of a child with a disability. Frequently, neither wants to burden the other with their pain; they are very protective of each other. Unfortunately, this can be misinterpreted as indifference. Grandparents can be mistakenly viewed as being cold and uninvolved when in reality they are frightened and concerned but diffident about sharing their feelings. The parents and grandparents often need help in bridging the gap between them.

In the Emerson College program, we always try to provide a support group for grandparents, usually the most isolated and loneliest family members. It is difficult to assemble enough grandparents to have a group because many of them now live long distances from their children and visit only intermittently. Nevertheless, we make the attempt every year by scheduling a nursery day on a Saturday—long in advance and in the spring when grandparents are more likely to return to the north—in the hope that we can gather enough grandparents for a group. I really enjoy a grandparent group, not only because I can relate so well to them because we are at similar life-cycle points, but also because of how lonely they are and how much they need support from us and from each other. These groups are invariably intense because for some grandparents, this is the first opportunity they have had to grieve openly.

Occasionally many of the grandparents in a nursery group live in our local area. When this happens, we offer the group an evening meeting in which I use the fishbowl design. Groups such as these almost invariably spark a great deal of family dialogue. They are also among the most professionally satisfying groups that I lead.

Occasionally we have dealt with families in which the grandparent are more capable than the parents and have assumed the primary caretaker role for a child with a disability. They do not respond in entirely the same way as parents of a child with a hearing impairment. For example, they do not take responsibility for the hearing loss. Their pain and guilt is usually due to concerns about their own child's perceived ineptitude and how they must have failed him or her. They must be given a chance to mourn this loss. I enjoy working with grandparents raising a grandchild with a hearing impairment because they are older and wiser, with a perspective that first-time parents do not have. They are also determined to not make the same mistakes they did with their own child.

After they have worked through their pain and anger, parents frequently discover that the child's grandparents are an important resource for them, although not in the way that they had originally expected. Grandparents frequently provide respite care via necessary babysitting so that parents can have some time out. Grandparents can also provide necessary parenting to the other siblings in the family when the parents are overwhelmed by the demands of the child with a disability. The surrogate parent role played by the grandparents can become very important for the emotional well-being of the nondisabled siblings. Once the parent gets through the existential crisis, the restructured relationship between him or her and the grandparents can also be very exciting. For the first time, the parents can begin to feel like, and respond as, adults with their own parents, who in turn find themselves being treated as adults.

Siblings

Siblings are enormously important for the development of social skills. Within the sibling system, children learn how to resolve conflicts and how to be supportive of one another. They learn how to make friends and allies, how to save face while losing, and how to achieve recognition for their skills. The sibling system teaches children to negotiate, cooperate, and compete. The jockeying for position within the family system shapes and molds children into their adult personas. When children come in contact with the world outside the family, they use the knowledge they learned from their siblings in forming their peer relationships (Minuchin, 1974).

The sibling relationship is potentially the longest relationship in our lifetime. In some families, this relationship is fostered and strong; in others, it is very weak. Siblings also serve to validate our experiences while growing up and are the closest thing we have to someone who shares our childhood experiences.

There is little in the literature about the effects of a child with a disability on the sibling system. Probably the most definitive study was done by Grossman (1972), who tested and interviewed 83 college students who had siblings with developmental delays. She found that 90% of the participants had been affected by their siblings who had the developmental delay. The 10% who were not affected were the oldest male children. The most affected were the oldest sisters, who were expected to participate in childrearing activities and to assume many parental functions. In most families, there are different role expectations for oldest sons and oldest daughters. All younger siblings were affected one way or another by the child with a mental disability. The effects on the siblings were both negative and positive; in fact, the study participants split evenly, with 45% feeling that overall it was a negative experience and 45% feeling that it was a positive one.

The following negative consequences were noted by Grossman:

1. shame about the child with the developmental delay, and guilt about that shame;

2. guilt about being in good health while the sibling was not;

3. a sense of being tainted or defective—concern that they themselves might have a mental disability or might bear children with a disability;

4. guilt about having negative feelings toward the sibling who has the disability;

5. a feeling of having been neglected by the parents;

6. a feeling of having lost their own childhood because of the too-early assumption of responsibilities; and

7. a belief that the child with the disability had put stress on the parental relationship, which negatively affected the rest of the family.

The positives consequences for the siblings were as follows:

1. greater understanding of people in general and people with disabilities in particular,

2. more compassion,

3. more appreciation of their own good health and intelligence,

4. more sensitivity to prejudice,

5. a sense that the experience had drawn the family together, and

6. a sense of vocational purpose and direction. (Many siblings become teachers of children with special needs.)

coping

As one might expect, Grossman (1972) found that the more open and comfortable the parents were in talking about and accepting the child's disability, the better able the nondisabled sibling was to deal with it. When the parents accepted the child with a disability, they tended to help the nondisabled child also come to a healthy acceptance. This finding has strong clinical implications for professionals working with children with disabilities because by working with the parents, as system theory would predict, they can also be working with the sibling system. The other finding that needs to be emphasized is that as tragic as having a child with a disability may be, it can and does have a very positive effect on some families and on the children within those families.

Seligman and Lobato (1983) and Lobato (1983) reviewed all of the studies done on the nondisabled siblings of children with special needs. They concluded that there is a differential effect and called for longitudinal and more-controlled studies. I fully concur with this finding. There are few studies of siblings within the field of communication disorders. All the studies I have found are within the field of deafness; one wonders how siblings of children with speech and language disorders fare. My experience would lead me to believe that there is no disorder-specific response and that all siblings will respond in pretty much the same way, depending on the cues they receive from their parents.

Schwirian (1976) interviewed 29 mothers of families in which there was a preschool child with a hearing impairment who had older siblings and 28 mothers of families with only nondisabled children. She found that older nondisabled siblings of children with hearing impairments had greater care responsibilities and fewer social activities than older siblings in the control group. Sisters had significantly higher childcare and overall responsibility scores than did brothers, again indicating the different role expectations that parents have for sons and daughters. A major procedural weakness of the Schwirian study is that she did not interview or test the siblings. Her data are only as good as the mothers' observations of their children's feelings and behavior. In some cases, this may not be very accurate.

Israelite (1986) tested 14 hearing female adolescents (mean age of 16 years 3 months) who were the older sisters of children with hearing impairments and a matched group of 14 adolescents who had nondisabled siblings. All the tests used were self-report questionnaires. Israelite found that the two groups differed significantly on only two traits: self-concept identity and social self. The results suggested that the hearing siblings defined themselves not only as individuals in their own right, but as sisters of children with hearing impairments.

Darius (1988) interviewed siblings of children with hearing impairments. Her data indicated that siblings from small families, especially those with only two children, are most at risk for social and emotional difficulty. Siblings who are of the same gender and who are within 2 years of age of the deaf sibling are also at risk. Her data supported the idea that how well the parents accepted and adapted to the deafness was the major variable in the siblings' acceptance.

For my book *Deafness in the Family* (Luterman, 1987), I interviewed some of the original families that had gone through the Emerson College program. In one family, the oldest daughter had become a speech–language pathologist in Hawaii. I wrote and asked her to write me of her experiences growing up with a deaf brother. I think her letter, printed below, poignantly illustrates the problems of the hearing sibling.

Dear Dr. Luterman:

I have been very busy this spring with work, my two special education classes that I am taking at the University of Hawaii, and the new group that I joined called Sign Express. It is a group of about 15 people who sign songs and put on performances to help educate others about sign language.

I am real excited about the book you are writing and I wish that I could have been there to talk with you when you went over to my family's house. I have a lot of feelings about Robert's deafness and how it has affected me. I have only told my mother some of my feelings because she gets upset or angry when I say how I felt when I was little. I don't know if it's because she thinks that I am saying that she was not a good mother to me, or why she gets upset.

I think when I was little, I had very mixed feelings. I felt very jealous of Robert, but I also felt very proud of him. I can remember feeling very neglected because I always thought that he got all of the attention from everybody. Of course, now I realize that my mother had to work with him more and it was all necessary, but I didn't understand that when I was little. I remember wishing that I was deaf for a while, thinking that then I would get more attention. I remember wishing that I would get sick and have to go into the hospital so that everyone would bring me presents and give me more attention. I even remember trying to break my arm by jumping out of my treehouse (which never happened). I have never told my mother any of this. But I never hated Robert. I guess the way I dealt with my jealousy was by deciding to work with deaf children when I grew up. I decided this ever since I used to go watch Robert at Emerson College through the one-way mirror with my mother. And here I am, a speech pathologist working at a school where the deaf total communication class is housed, and I love working with the deaf kids (ages 5–12).

I also remember being very proud of Robert. I can remember going to his school plays at the school for the deaf and having tears come to my eyes when I watched him on stage. I remember wanting to be friends with his friends there. I also remember people saying mean things about deaf people in general, like they can't talk and they are all "deaf and dumb," and feeling so hurt and intimidated that I couldn't even stand up for deaf people. I usually just said nothing.

I guess Robert's deafness probably created a lot of extra tension in my parents' marriage. I remember my mother getting really upset about the taxis taking him to school, some school problem, and other things. I remember my father not wanting or just not getting involved and my mother getting upset at him. I really never understood just how it affected my father, but I know it was real hard on my mother. I never really noticed what effect Robert's deafness had on Lynda, Michael, or Nicole [siblings]. I didn't get along with Lynda, Michael, or Robert that much when I was little. Now I am much closer to everyone in my family.

Maybe it's because I live so far away [that] I am trying to learn to sign fluently. Robert prefers to sign now and doesn't associate with hearing people if he can help it. Last summer when I went home for a visit, I played the card game Uno with Robert and his friends. At first I felt uncomfortable, but it was a lot of fun and I think that was the first time anyone in our family associated with him when he had his friends over. I wish I could spend more time with him and really get to know him. I have been able to get a hold of a TTY a few times, and I love being able to talk to him over the phone. I always felt bad when I called home on holidays and could talk to everyone and then just be able to tell someone to say hi to Robert. I remember a couple of times he would get on the phone to say hi to me and then my mother would get on the phone and say "that was Robert," like I couldn't tell. I remember when we used to watch TV when we were little and Robert would always ask us what was going on in the show and we would get irritated at him and tell him to wait for the commercials. I wish we knew how to sign then and be able to interpret for him so he could understand while the show was on. I have very strong feelings about total communication. Robert has told me a lot about how he always felt left out, and that makes me feel so sad for him because if we only used sign language he would have been more involved and would have known what was going on. But I realize that is a big issue that probably never will be solved.

Well I guess I rambled on quite a bit. I hope that this information will be helpful to you. If you have any more questions, please feel free to write to me. I'll be glad to help in any way possible. I would love to visit you the next time I get back to Boston and also visit the clinic at Emerson College.

Thank you for asking [about] my feelings.

How often do we ask siblings how they feel or include them in what we do? They can be immensely helpful in conducting diagnostics and in administering therapy. I often use them as test models for their sibling with the hearing impairment. In the nursery program, we always set aside several days each semester specifically for siblings. On these days, the hearing children are allowed into the nursery and the therapy sessions. We give them a hearing test so that they know what takes place in a test suite. We are always very careful to ask them if there is something they want to know. Very often the siblings are our future speech pathologists and audiologists.

At some point, all parent groups in which I have participated have brought up the problem of siblings. It often occurs in the first meeting because parents have been burdened by the guilty knowledge that they have been ignoring the hearing sibling in the family. The solution to the sibling problem is easy to grasp intellectually and very hard to implement practically.

Parents need to direct attention to the sibling as a person, not merely as a vehicle to produce a well-functioning child with a disability or as an impediment to that mission. Means must be found within the family for the sharing of feelings, and siblings must be given a chance to discuss their feelings of anger and guilt. Unfortunately, a fair balance is not easy to achieve, especially in the early years, because the parents do not have much energy and time for themselves, let alone for the nondisabled siblings. Parents frequently can identify the problem; however, because of limited resources, they cannot implement a solution. In this situation, the grandparents can be very helpful. Also, paradoxically, if we can teach parents to take care of themselves, they will have the energy and time left to share with the nondisabled siblings. Parents don't always see that it is not the quantity of time they spend as much as it is the quality.

Parents, siblings & grandparents working together

Optimal Families

When we broaden our view from individual therapy to family therapy, as proposed in this text, we in effect become a member of the family, and as a member of the family, we teach by modeling effective behavior. For us to do this, we need to have a grasp of what it is we are working toward to help the family become more optimal. Several models of the optimal family have appeared in the family literature (Beavers & Voeller, 1983; Epstein, Bishop, & Baldwin, 1982; Olson, Russell, & Sprenkle, 1983). From these studies, I have distilled five characteristics of the optimal family.

1. Communication among all family members is clear and direct. Almost any family therapist who has written about families has examined their internal communication patterns. Invariably, dysfunctional families have dysfunctional communication patterns. Using modeling, therapists encourage clear communication. Optimal families do not hold back or talk around an issue. Implicit expectations are always made explicit; comments are always directed toward the person for whom they are intended; talking is efficient and straightforward; and messages are congruent, containing both content and feelings. Empathy and humor characterize the communication among family members.

2. Roles and responsibilities are clearly delineated, overlapping, and flexible. An optimal family must have clear intergenerational boundaries, as well as a delineated sibling subsystem. The parents must have clear authority over other roles, which are allocated on the basis of ability rather than on the basis of age or gender. Roles need to be overlapping as well so that if one member of the family is not present, others can fill in. The children's responsibilities need to be altered as they grow, and responsibilities need to be renegotiated periodically. There must be a basis and structure for negotiation of role allocation. Optimal families allow for change in roles as needed to maintain a well-functioning unit.

3. The family members accept limits for the resolution of conflict. Conflict in families is normal and healthy; growth and change come about as a result of conflict. Parent–child and sibling relationships are inherently conflictual. In dysfunctional families, conflict is repressed; the family might appear harmonious, but when conflict does emerge, it becomes destructive. In optimal families, disputes are resolved in a way that is mutually satisfactory, and there is always a face-saving formula for any "loser." Conflict in an optimal family usually involves everyone winning. For example, the mother is about to cut a cake and the children are squabbling over who is going to get the bigger piece. The mother lets one child cut the cake and the other child choose the first slice; the next time, the second child will cut the cake and the first child will choose. Children need to see that solutions are fair and that individual needs are always considered. Parents must also model conflict resolution for their children as the professionals modeled it for them. For humans, eventual success as a species depends on finding and maintaining good conflict-resolution skills. These skills develop first within a family context and are then extended to society.

4. Intimacy is prevalent and is a function of frequent, equal-powered transactions. One basic function of the family is to provide an environment where members feel loved. Families have different ways of expressing love: Some express it physically through hugging and kissing, whereas others use more subtle expressions of caring. The caring needs to be communicated in a way that the other family members can receive. An optimal family provides intimacy while also respecting the need for space and distance. Optimal families are cohesive without being enmeshed and stifling.

5. A healthy balance exists between change and the maintenance of stability. The maintenance of stability is known as *homeostasis*. Families maintain their balance by making minute adjustments, much as a high-wire performer oscillates movements to stay on the wire (Harvey, 1989). Families must change to accommodate the life cycle. For example, as children age, they place new demands on the parents' system of restrictions. Meanwhile the parents are aging and are less adept at managing their lives, so other family members must fill the void. Then there are the vicissitudes of life when a family is thrown a "curve ball." This happens when parents get ill; when an economic catastrophe, such as the loss of a job, occurs; or when a child is born with a disability. Optimal families are able to make the necessary adjustments while maintaining stability. Dysfunctional families are not able to accommodate to the change and often dissolve or become so dysfunctional that they need massive amounts of external support.

The delicate balance between homeostasis and accommodating to change involves all of the other factors involved in an optimal family. Change can be accomplished best where there is open and clear communication among the family members and where role flexibility enables others to step in to accommodate the increased demands on family time. Family members need to care about each other, and the family needs to have a means of dealing with the conflict that is inevitable any time there is a need for change.

Optimal families produce optimally functioning children and adults with disabilities. Our job as professionals in working with persons with communication disorders is to help the family become optimal or as close to it as possible. Through modeling, we can teach parents how to manage conflict, communicate openly and honestly with their children, and display their affection and caring for their children. In effect, what we must do is parent the parents and create for them in our relationship an optimal family. The parents can then take from our optimal clinical family the information and skills necessary for their own home situation.

The Successful Family

The idea of the optimal family is basically theoretical, stemming from the experience of family therapists working with dysfunctional families; however, some research on the successful family does exist. The design of these studies was basically the same: Professionals working with the families rated their degree of success in coping with a child with a disability. Based on the ratings, the investigators then categorized families as successful, adequate, or inadequate. These families were then interviewed to determine the characteristics that led to the professional judgment. Gallagher et al. (1981) examined families in which there was a child with developmental delay, Lavell and Keogh (1980) examined families in which there was a child with diabetes, and Venters (1981) studied families in which there was a child with cystic fibrosis. The results of these studies suggest that four characteristics seem to underlie a successful family. These characteristics are very much in agreement with my own observations of the families of children who are deaf.

1. A successful family is one that feels empowered. Families need to feel that what they are doing will make a difference. Even with children who have cystic fibrosis, a terminal illness, the parents need to feel that by working with the children, they can prolong their lives and make their current lives easier. I frequently see professionals who present such a bleak and hopeless picture to these parents that the parents never get over the feeling of "What's the use." These families are never successful. We must never take away hope.

Parents are often rendered impotent by too much help from professionals. Sandow and Clarke (1977) studied the effects of a home intervention program on the performance of preschool children with severe down syndrome and severe cerebral palsy. The 32 children in the study were divided into two matched groups. One group was visited by a therapist once every 2 weeks for a 2-hour session, whereas the other group was visited only once every 2 months. The study was conducted for 3 years, and at the end of each year the children were tested for their cognitive functioning and speech and language development. The findings were startling. Initially, the more frequently visited children showed more gains in intellectual functioning and growth in speech and language than did the less frequently visited children. By the second year of the study, the results had reversed, with the less frequently visited children demonstrating more improvement than the more frequently visited children. By the third year, the gap had increased even further, demonstrating that less professional intervention was better than more. The researchers interpreted their data to suggest that parents in the less frequently visited group were less dependent on the therapist than were the more frequently visited parents. In short, the parents became empowered because they were forced to rely on their own skills and strengths due to a minimum amount of professional help.

My bias concerning home intervention programs is that they should be almost entirely parent centered and that the teachers should interact minimally with the child. The parent should do the lesson, and the teacher should focus on those things that the parent is doing well. The help provided by the teacher to the parent needs to be covert and not very apparent if the parent is to be empowered.

2. In successful families the self-esteem, especially of the mother, is high. This notion is very much related to the empowering notion discussed above. I think that the single most potent clinical intervention we can make to help a young client with a disability is to bolster the self-esteem of the parents, especially that of the mother. There is research justification for this idea. In a hallmark study, Schlessinger (1994) followed 40 families with a deaf child on a longitudinal basis for 20 years. She found that the best predictor of third-grade literacy was the self-esteem of the parents. This variable transcended hearing loss, methodology, and socioeconomic status. This means that every clinical intervention that we perform needs to be evaluated in terms of whether or not it enhances the self-esteem of the parents. The efficacy of our clinical interventions is going to be a matter of parental self-esteem.

When parents feel confident and empowered, they no longer need denial as a coping strategy, and then they are able to work with the professional as coequals. When this happens, the child benefits immensely. In the same way, when working with adult clients, professional attention needs to be directed at empowering and increasing the self-confidence of the nondisabled spouse.

Therapists need to set up situations whereby the parents can experience some success in working with their children, especially in the early stages of the parent–professional interaction. As Featherstone (1980) so eloquently stated, "Fears ease as experience discredits fantasy, as mothers and fathers learn that actual problems of raising their child differ from the ones they imagined. Similarly, small victories over private demons reassure parents about their own ability to raise their child" (p. 27).

3. In successful families there is a feeling that the burden is shared. In most families, one person—usually the mother or the nondisabled spouse—is designated as the primary caretaker and therapist for the person with a disability. If the rest of the family provides no support and respite care, the designated caregiver begins to feel resentful. When this happens, there is very little likelihood of a successful outcome. Other family members need not be overt in their help, but they need to be emotionally supportive of the caretaker and also be willing to assume some of the other family responsibilities, thus freeing the caretaker to provide the direct therapy. This can occur even in a single-parent home if there is a supportive network around the primary caretaker. Friends and other family members can fill in for the missing parent. Dundon, Carmer, and Novak (1987) found that two major variables determining the success of families in coping with Alzheimer's disease were health of the well spouse and the amount of unpaid help available to the family—when the well spouse felt supported by the community, the family coped successfully

The family also needs to feel that the larger community is supportive and is sharing the burden. In the initial diagnostic stages when the client is a young child, the parents feel totally responsible. I often tell them, "This business is really in thirds—one third is your responsibility, one third is mine as a professional, and one third is the child's. You just be sure that you do your third, I'll do my third, and both of us will see that the child does his or her third."

4. Successful families need to make philosophical sense of the situation. All of us have a cosmology that is our way of explaining why and how things happen, especially why bad things happen. Because it is hard for most of us to accept the existential notion of randomness or the concept that we live in a world without meaning, we seek an answer to the question, "Why me?" To not have a suitable answer may leave us stuck in bitterness and anger, which seldom lead to a successful outcome. Each family must come up with its own answer, which means that we as professionals sometimes need to get into uncomfortable areas of discussion as people come to grips with their own explanation of why the terrible thing happened to them. For example, in one support group, a parent of a deaf child said, "Since this happened, I have stopped going to church," and a mother sitting opposite her said, "Since this happened, I've been going to church every day." A very fruitful discussion then ensued, as the parents worked through their feelings toward God and reworked their religious views.

A very successful mother of two children who are deaf and one child who has severe brain damage as a result of a car accident had this to say at a group counseling session:

> I always think of myself as a very average person. I have no particular talent, no particular anything. I'm a very average type person, and I've been given three very special kids. Sometimes I talk to God and I say, "Why did you give these kids to me? Why didn't you give them to someone who was different?" and so then I think, "All right, I was given these kids and maybe this is my thing in life. Maybe all I'm going to do in life is to get these kids into adulthood, and maybe this is how my salvation will be measured."

With an explanation we can move toward and work; without one, we are forever pondering the why. Having a wife with multiple sclerosis challenged me to make something good happen out of an awful disease. There is a marvelous Zen saying, "When the learner is ready, the teacher appears." For me and my wife, multiple sclerosis was our teacher.

The stress on families, which is both a reflection of sociological changes and the change engendered by a person with a disability, is not necessarily a negative force. I have seen a great deal of growth occur as a result of this stress. Many siblings decide to become therapists. Although some marriages founder, others are strengthened. For parents, the child with a disability can offer an opportunity to restructure a relationship that has gone stale. Men have often reported how delighted they were to find out how much strength their wives have; the wives were delighted with the caring qualities that emerged in their husbands. Often both parents have found a new purpose in working hard together in parent organizations and therapy programs, thereby strengthening the bond between them.

Similarly, the parent–grandparent relationship can be restructured. For the first time, many parents begin to respond as adults to their own parents and in time find themselves being treated as adults. They often begin to see their own parents as vulnerable fellow adults, and that is very exciting.

I have always found growth in stress. I am pushed by the stress to develop more capacity in order to reduce the stress. We generally give to life what life demands. When life demands more, I am forced to expand. That increased capacity is my growth. I see this happening in all the families with whom I have worked, and although I can empathize and perhaps sympathize with the pain involved, I know that if they can just hang on, they will learn and grow. We professionals must allow the process of growth to take place. We can facilitate it by not overhelping and at all times respecting our clients dignity and their capacity to grow. Very often we have to let go of our preconceived notions. The following anonymously written poem has helped me with this:

To Let Go

> To Let Go is not to stop caring,
> It's recognizing I can't do it for someone else.
> To Let Go is not to cut myself off,
> It's realizing I can't control another.
> To Let Go is not to enable,
> But to allow learning from natural consequences.
> To Let Go is not to fight Powerlessness,
> But to accept the outcome is not in my hands.
>
> To Let Go is not to try to change or blame others,
> It's to make the most of myself.

To Let Go is not to care for, it's to care about.
To Let Go is not to fix, it's to be supportive.
To Let Go is not to judge,
It's to allow another to be a human being.
To Let Go is not to try to arrange outcomes,
But to allow others to affect their own destinies.

To Let Go is not to be protective,
It's to permit another to face their own reality.
To Let Go is not to regulate anyone,
But to strive to become what I dream I can be.

To Let Go is not to fear less, it's to love more.

CHAPTER

COUNSELING AND THE FIELD OF COMMUNICATION DISORDERS

Educating the Clinician

During the 1960s, a notable attempt was made to define the fields of speech–language pathology and audiology by giving them a narrow, technical base. This ensured survival as independent professions with a solid core of research expertise and scientific credibility. Now that these fields are established, the move has been toward more humanistic, family-oriented fields that borrow heavily from psychology, social work, and family therapy.

It presently appears that training programs are lagging behind the fields' needs. As stated in Chapter 1, McCarthy et al. (1986) conducted a survey of the ASHA-accredited training programs. They found that only 40% of these programs offered a course in counseling within their department, 36% offered a course outside the department (more than half of these courses were offered within psychology and education departments and had no content related to speech and hearing), and 23% offered no course in counseling. Only one third of the programs required that students take a counseling course, despite the fact that 70% of the respondents felt that counseling was a very important skill that should be offered within the program. The authors concluded their study with the following observation:

> Although the fields of audiology and speech–language pathology recognize counseling as an essential component of diagnostic and therapeutic

procedures and as a professional responsibility, the emphasis training programs place on it may not reflect its importance. Students are often trained in counseling theory and techniques only when they have chosen to take such a course. Even then, counseling specific to communication disorders is frequently not included. These data are underscored by the finding that only 12% of the respondents in this study felt that training programs are sufficiently preparing students to meet the counseling needs of individuals with communicative disorders. (p. 52)

The follow up to that study indicated no essential change (Culpepper et al., 1994) and was further reinforced by Rosenberg's (1997) finding that 82% of 435 surveyed speech–language pathology graduate students felt they needed more counseling practicum experience. I also believe that we are not training our students appropriately to prepare them to meet the emotional demands of helping professions. From the humanistic point of view, a client's learning and growth take place best in a nonthreatening atmosphere of warmth and acceptance. In order to facilitate this growth, the therapist needs to be a caring, nonjudgmental, congruent person. None of these skills is exotic; they are all within the purview of everyone. The job of the training program is to help develop these attributes in student clinicians. Unfortunately, almost all graduate training programs tend to stress the intellectual and cognitive skills of the students, not their interpersonal abilities. For example, selection of students is generally based on the intellectual skills exemplified by Graduate Record Examination scores or grade-point averages. Rarely are interpersonal skills considered, except perhaps indirectly as reflected in letters of recommendation; however, the present era of full disclosure and threats of litigation has rendered letters of recommendation almost meaningless. The grade-point average seems to lend an objective measure that we can defend. Interpersonal skills are not readily measurable and may be difficult to defend if challenged by an irate student. Ignoring interpersonal skills, however, is very dangerous; we can turn out students who are knowledgeable but clinically and interpersonally inept.

It appears that we are selecting reasonably "normal" graduate students. Crane and Cooper (1983) gave the Minnesota Multiphasic Personality Inventory (MMPI; Lachar, n.d.) to 130 women speech–language graduate students. They found that the resultant profiles "were manifestly normal but rather passive, compliant, stereotypically feminine, sensitive, anxious" (p. 139). It concerns me that we are willing to accept these attributes as "normal" for women. I prefer to think that much of what we are viewing as "stereotypically feminine" is in reality a reflection of our teaching and attitudes toward women. I hope that this attitude is changing. I am deeply concerned about the passivity and compliance aspects of the personality profile and what that bodes for our profession.

In all fairness, Crane and Cooper also found that these students were highly imaginative, creative, and energetic—and I have certainly met and worked with my share of students with these delightful characteristics. From the research of Miller and Potter (1982), however, we also know that many of these students will burn out at an alarming rate.

Training Students for Clinical Competence and Personal Growth

I am not sure that the MMPI measures some important personality variables that influence clinical competency. For example, the Annie Sullivan type of student needs to be identified early in his or her career. This is a caring person with energy and a marvelous impulse to be helpful that can be directed, but we must provide experiences at the training level to bolster self-esteem and increase self-awareness of the need to be needed. The Annie Sullivan types must learn how to help in a way that is truly useful so that the client's self-esteem and independence are not compromised. Our personal satisfactions can come from knowing internally what we have done and not from receiving the approval of others. In short, we have to help develop in students an inner locus of evaluation and not leave them field-dependant for approval.

Occasionally we get interpersonally inept students who are otherwise quite bright, and there needs to be a place within our profession for them. I think they can become more adept with some structured interpersonal experiences; they may also make good researchers.

Occasionally our screening process fails to identify another kind of student: the individual with a very limited capacity to care for others. These are students who are very self-focused, and who in psychological jargon would be described as narcissistic. I think that I can teach almost anything except the capacity to care. These students probably will be professional disasters despite any technical skills we might teach them, and we need to have better mechanisms to screen such students out of the profession.

If one examines closely the training of speech–language pathologists and audiologists, it becomes apparent that it is developed along poorly conceived behavioral lines. Control is generally external to the students: The teacher decides what the students need to know and rewards them if they appear to learn the material. Student clinicians also learn to please the supervisor, which also encourages the development of an external locus of evaluation. (No wonder they are passive and compliant!) How often do students get a chance to select material to be learned, and how often are they required to evaluate themselves and, perhaps, their supervisor?

The communication disorders literature reveals a strong humanistic trend in the supervisory relationship. Ward and Webster (1965) urged that we as teachers treat our students as human beings and that their self-actualization be an important consideration in the training program. They argued for courses within the curriculum that are geared to explain human behaviors and that can then be applied to students. Van Riper (1965), a pioneer in speech–language pathology, described so aptly the sometimes painful role of the supervisor:

> He is a friendly person looking on interestedly in what is taking place, warmly empathizing with the success and making no issue about the failures. Even when the student is demonstrating outrageous sins of omission or commission, the supervisor does not seize the reins. He suffers silently and keeps a poker face and formulates what he will say to the clinician later. (p. 77)

Van Riper believed that we should treat the student clinician with the same loving respect that we wish him or her to accord the client.

Pickering (1977) argued that the student needs to have relationship skills as much as field knowledge. According to Pickering, the supervisory relationship can be the vehicle for the student to learn about relationships and for promoting personal growth and change in both the supervisor and student. This relationship needs to have the elements of authenticity, dialogue, risk taking, and conflict in order to facilitate growth.

Caracciolo et al. (1978) wrote that a supervisor should model the Rogerian nondirective role, which has a high degree of unconditional regard, empathy, and congruence. After experiencing growth through this humanistic relationship with the supervisor, the students in turn would be able to foster this kind of relationship with their clients.

I agree with Caracciolo et al.'s (1978) premise that experiencing the humanistic relationship is the best way of learning it. The authors made me uncomfortable, however, when they stated that "it is necessary to define operationally and construct specific training procedures that will develop among supervisors the necessary attitudes and skills that will contribute to personal and professional growth" (p. 290). It seems to me that when we set about "operationally defining" and "developing specific training procedures," we lose the essence of the humanistic approach and have moved into a behavioral model. At some fundamental level, humanism is ineffable. True learning is an inside-out process; we must lead students to it and hope they find it by creating for them the conditions of a growth-promoting relationship. When we deliberately structure the learning situation to teach techniques, we are imposing a cognitive solution on an affect problem, and our students tend to learn the form of the approach but not its substance. (Anyone who has tried to have a conversation with a student who thinks that Rogerian reflective listening means repeating back the last thing the person has said begins to get an insight into the causes of homicide.)

Klevans, Volz, and Friedman (1981) attempted to train students in interpersonal skills. One experimental group was taught skills via extended role playing in an out-of-class assignment in which group members had to assume the role of a person with a speech, language, or hearing impairment. The second group was required to observe clinical interactions and to code behavior. The authors found that the students in the experiential group were able to make significantly more facilitative verbal responses than the observing/coding group when tested in a simulated helping relationship. The authors also noted that the length of time (8 3/4 hours) devoted to training both groups was insufficient for mastering interpersonal skills.

I think this study points out several things that need to be examined. If we are going to train students in interpersonal skills, the experience needs to be hands-on rather than didactic. We cannot lecture within a class or even have students observe interactions and then expect them to be interpersonally adept. It is also clear that we have to allot more time within the curriculum for working on interpersonal skills. The $8\frac{3}{4}$ hours of time allotted in this study, which was part of a 1-credit clinic practice course, is unfortunately typical of most training programs and rather pathetic for attempting to teach such fundamental clinical skills.

Recently, English, Mendel Rajeski, and Hornak (1999) demonstrated that listening behavior and making affect responses could be taught to graduate students in audiology who were enrolled in a counseling course. This study also used a structured activity that was perhaps useful to the future clinicians but may not have gone far enough.

I think we also need to attack the problem from the personal growth side. We cannot limit our endeavors to teaching interpersonal skills from a strictly technique point of view. For me, the best way of teaching and learning counseling has been within the context of my own personal growth experiences, which have included such diverse activities as attendance at workshops, immersion in sensitivity groups, and an Outward Bound learning experience where I had to rock climb and sail. Especially helpful was the last experience, which had an underlying theme of "We have met the enemy and found it is us." More recently it has been with yoga and meditation. Every year I look for experiences that will further my personal growth. I have found that as I have come to accept myself more, I have also accepted and valued others more. I have had to learn to give myself permission to think, feel, and be productive, and I need to bring that element of self to the teacher–student relationship.

The dilemma of the supervisory/teaching relationship in developing humanistic relationships with students is the evaluative function held by the teacher. As long as the supervisor/teacher has the power of the grade, locus of control is always external to the student and authenticity on the student's part in relation to the supervisor is hard to accomplish. At some level and at some time, the student must please the teacher in order to get a passing grade. It would require a high degree of trust to develop authenticity in the relationship. True equality is not really possible because the levels of personal power are inherently unequal. Van Riper (1965) argued that we should be collaborators with our students rather than supervisors, an ideal that is very hard to accomplish when the supervisors must give the students grades or eventually write letters of recommendation. Although the supervisors may believe that they are collaborators, the students feel differently. Culatta, Colucci, and Wiggins (1975), for example, found wide discrepancies between the supervisors' and the student clinicians' views of their relationship.

In my teaching of content-level courses, I have attempted to work out a compromise between cognitive and interpersonal learning needs. At the beginning of the course, I give the students the final examination, which consists of a list of essay questions that reflect my opinion about what content they need to master and from which I will select some unspecified number of questions. I also give the students a bibliography containing readings that will enable them to find the answers to the questions. It is then the students' responsibility to organize their time to master that content. The grade for the course is based solely on the examination performance, and students are encouraged to be as ignorant as possible during class sessions. I comment that they should be ignorant—that's why they are taking the course. The only time they cannot afford to be ignorant is on the final examination.

I usually take responsibility for structuring half of the class sessions with lectures, films, videos, or guest speakers; the students are required to structure the other half. These latter halves usually start out with painful silences until the students realize that nothing happens until they make it happen. Periodically we evaluate the class, and everyone, including myself, has a chance to talk about how things are going. Within this format, the students get a chance to obtain some control over what they learn; they have to take responsibility for obtaining content and are never required to read anything. Generally students' course evaluations are enthusiastic, although as we near examination time, their anxiety begins to increase and they regret their freedom. Because the students are not usually familiar with a learning situation in which they have to assume so much responsibility, they frequently use their time to meet the demands of other courses and, as a result, find themselves far behind in our course. Bargaining sessions frequently ensue in which they try to limit the scope of the examination, delay the final, and so on. I delight in the give-and-take of the negotiations in which we engage, as it reflects an equality and an authenticity in our relationship. I generally remain tough; if the students are to learn responsibility assumption, they must not be let off the responsibility hook lightly.

My sense of teaching this way is that the students get as much, and often more, content than they did when I took sole responsibility for it. I also am astonished at the interesting byways of content that emerge out of the students' interests. For example, a recent aural rehabilitation class decided to read the play *Children of a Lesser God*, which describes the relationship between a woman who is deaf and a hearing male speech therapist. From the in-class play reading and discussion, the students obtained a great deal of insight into the problems of deaf–hearing relationships and of contemporary issues among adults who are deaf. This understanding was of a much deeper dimension than they would have obtained from a review of the didactic literature alone.

Evidence in the literature suggests that locus of control can be shifted to a more internal orientation as a result of learning or teaching experiences. Johnson and Croft (1975) found that students enrolled in a personalized system of instruction (PSI) course demonstrated a statistically significant internally oriented shift as measured by the Rotter scale after they had completed the course. The PSI course had no midterm or final examination; it was entirely self-paced and self-graded, and performance was often evaluated in a personal interview. This sort of course can be modified to become a marvelous blend of behaviorist and humanist notions. Similarly based courses, which would include more contact with the teacher within a humanistic relationship, could be developed within the field of communication disorders in order to develop self-managing students who also have experienced a clinically and personally useful relationship with a teacher.

In these professionally perilous times of high burnout rates and declining student enrollment, we must find creative solutions to implementing a humanistic-based education that encourages an inner locus of control. This is not to say that we should give up our cognitive and evaluative functions; instead, we must supplement content with interpersonal learning. It is unreasonable to expect students trained within the current poorly conceived behavioral model to easily take responsibility for themselves or for their profession. The behavioral model, with its emphasis on external locus of control and external locus of evaluation, tends to produce professionals who will accept poor working conditions, work mechanically, and not take responsibility for furthering the profession by passively and compliantly accepting things as they are. If we do not anticipate change and act, we will be overwhelmed by it. I believe that the futures of speech–language pathology and audiology rest in altering current educational practices to include a more humanistic base that will in turn create a more self-confident, self-reliant, and assertive professional—one who will also be much more effective in serving persons with communication disorders.

Training Students for Parent Programs

If there is going to be any meaningful change in the current parent–professional relationship, it will have to occur at the professional training level. Too many young clinicians leave their training programs with minimal or very inadequate experience in relating to parents. I suspect that part of the problem lies in the lack of practice in working with parents of the supervisors and academic teachers in their training programs. The new ASHA regulations allow only 25 clock hours of student activity with parents to be counted toward the 375 hours needed for certification. Cartwright and Ruscello (1979) suggested that 10% of the total student contact hours with parents be allowed to count for certification, which seems quite reasonable to me.

On a national level, we also need to promote continuing education workshops specifically geared toward professionals in academic programs on the use of parents and the training of students in parental involvement. We need to increase the number and quality of our parental involvement programs throughout the nation. Only half of all approved clinics have such a program (Cartwright & Ruscello, 1979). This figure seems inadequate to me, especially because nearly 90% of all programs report that parental involvement is very important. We should also be very concerned about the quality of the existing parent programs. There are too many professional-centered parent programs (i.e., programs in which the professional has the control and uses the educational program to promote a particular point of view) in which the personal growth of the parents is minimal. A good parent program has to be designed with the parent in mind. If we try to append a parent program onto an existing child-centered program, we are doomed to failure. The program rapidly becomes the PTA model of parent involvement, which usually entails hurried parent conferences and lectures in which parents are talked at rather than listened to. In good programming, the parent is the primary target.

Good parent programs have a "snowball effect." They produce self-confident, positively-assertive parents who will work as equals with other professionals. These parents, in effect, become trainers of all professionals.

They open the eyes of professionals to the potential of parental involvement. The reasonably self-confident professional finds it a relief to have a parent as a coworker.

If parent–professional relationships are to improve, they have to be freed from a problem-centered orientation. Much of the contact between parent and professional occurs only when there is a specific problem. It is very hard to have a productive relationship when it is always problem-centered. I give my aural rehabilitation class a role-playing situation in which a teacher of students who are deaf calls a parent to school to tell the parent that his or her child is "an oral failure" and should be put in a total communication program. The problem is set up to be adversarial in that the parent is strongly committed to an oral education. The situation usually ends up in disaster. If this is the first parent–professional meeting (as generally happens), it is already too late; time has not been spent in developing the necessary trust, autonomy, and initiative that is necessary for dealing with such a loaded topic as changing the mode of communication for the child.

Some of my students solve this problem well. They recognize that the person with the problem is the teacher, not the parent or the child. When the teacher can convey to the parent that the teacher has a problem and can enlist the parent's help, then the relationship does not become adversarial. Both parent and teacher can embark together on a quest to find the best way of educating the child. It is also agreed by the class after the role-playing activity that the teacher should have seen the parents outside of the school and established and worked on their relationship before any problems occurred.

Parents and professionals in speech–language pathology are natural allies. They both want the same thing: a child with better communicating skills. In an almost lyrically written and lovely book on parents called *Special Children, Special Parents*, Murphy (1981), wrote, "Parents and workers are sculptors helping to shape what a child may become. There is a place for all—a place to be, to become something more than they now are, a place to learn, to dance, to sing" (p. ix).

Professional Burnout

The problem of professional burnout in the helping professions is quite severe. Meadow (1981) administered a burnout inventory to 240 teachers of persons who are deaf, and among the findings of her study were the following:

- Teachers of the deaf had a higher burnout rate than classroom teachers who were teaching children with normal hearing.

- Burnout was highest among teachers who had been working 7 to 10 years in the job and was lowest among teachers who had been working 11 or more years and among new teachers.

- Burnout was directly related to perceived ability to influence the work situation. Teachers who felt they had the power to influence their jobs displayed the least burnout.

- Teachers who had the highest personal involvement in their jobs also tended to have the highest burnout rate.

These results are very interesting. Greater stress appears to occur among professionals working with persons with disabilities than among professionals working with nondisabled populations. Young teachers seem to be carried through their first years by idealism and enthusiasm. From the Meadow (1981) data and from my own observations it appears that many young beginning teachers get overinvolved with the children with whom they are working. Mattingly (1977) noticed this phenomenon among childcare workers: Burnout was signaled by workers who began to merge themselves and their lives with the institution. When this merging occurred, the individual lost the resources he or she needed to be able to give to others. A helping professional is very much like a gasoline station where people come to fill up. At some point, a truck comes and fills the tanks of the gasoline station. The professional who merges with the population he or she is serving has little opportunity to "fill his or her own tank." I believe that this type of person is the most likely to burnout within that 7- to 10-year period.

Those professionals who survive beyond the 10-year period learn better coping strategies, probably because they have learned to meet their personal needs outside of their work experiences. From the Meadow (1981) data, it would also seem that they have a more internal locus of control than do the burnout sufferers, because burnout is directly related to the perceived inability to influence the work situation. Teachers with an inner locus of control are not "pushed into" accepting poor working conditions and are also more likely to assert themselves with administrators.

Within the context and terminologies of this book, burnout can be viewed as primarily a problem in dealing with the existential issue of loneliness and love: The need to be loved can push the teacher into an unwholesome, overinvolved relationship with his or her students. If we apply the Erikson model, we can also view burnout as an intimacy issue in that there is a fusion of the personal life and the job. Overall, I think that burnout is a locus-of-control problem because people who feel that they have no power, who are like "leaves in the wind," simply meeting other people's demands, will lose all feeling for their clients and will become emotionally exhausted and drained.

I think that we can effect changes in the burnout phenomenon by providing ongoing workshops and inservice training for working professionals. A more efficient way of dealing with this problem is to produce students who value themselves, who have an awareness of their own needs, who have an ability to be authentic in relationships, and who have more internal loci of control and evaluation.

Counseling Within the Public Schools

The public school setting is a difficult milieu for counseling to occur. The typical therapy model for the public school setting is one in which the children are taken out of class for individual therapy. Because of caseload numbers, therapists sometimes offer therapy in small groups. Contact with the parents is usually minimal, very often via a phone call and more often simply through messages carried back and forth by the child. It has always struck me that the underlying assumptions of this therapy model are incredibly naive. It assumes, in effect, that by working in isolation with the child for 1 hour a week (in some cases for only half an hour), a therapist can significantly alter the child's communication skills. It presupposes an incredibly powerful effect of individual therapy. Therapists who adopt this pull out model doom themselves to failure by working in a context that is not likely to succeed. It also burdens the child to be the change agent for the whole family system.

I think many therapists in the public schools intuitively recognize the absurdity of their professional lives. The restrictions they have accepted, either because those restrictions have been externally imposed or because of an internal reluctance to risk changing them, do not allow the therapists to do an effective job. When that happens, they either leave their jobs quickly or they burn out and go through the motions of the job, knowing full well that they are being ineffective.

There are ways to restructure jobs so that therapists become effective change agents. They need to see themselves as consultants/counselors rather than as direct purveyors of therapy. Where possible, therapy needs to be directed at the parents in order to be more effective. Within the public school setting, the teachers have the parental role. We can be much more efficient if we alter the classroom environment, which is the child's home away from home, so that it becomes more facilitative for the development of good communication skills for all the children. This means we must spend our time with the teachers in the classroom, helping them to help the children with communication disorders.

I think this consultative model of speech–language pathology is slowly taking hold and will become the dominant therapeutic model of the new millennium. Superior and Leichook (1986) strongly recommended a parent/consultant model within the public school setting. They suggested that "parent meetings could be scheduled in lieu of the child's treatment sessions, providing that the goal of parent consultation be addressed within the individual education plan. A few parent meetings may, in fact, have far greater effect than several therapy sessions" (p. 402). My sense is that the time spent with parents or teachers is usually the most fruitful time and that the thrust of therapy needs to be at the teacher/parent level.

In setting up the consultation model, it is critical that the therapist, before initiating any direct therapy with the child, meet with the classroom teachers and the child's parents. At this time, a clear contract needs to be drawn up that specifies everyone's expectations. I think the therapist needs to create a contract with the parents and the teachers that requires them to have some direct involvement in the therapeutic process. The contract has to be flexible, and opportunities must be provided for renegotiation. If there is any failure to meet contractual expectations, then the teacher/parent has to be "called on the carpet." It is absolutely essential that a working relationship be established before the initiation of therapy because it becomes the basis for any ongoing disputes involving the child or the contractual obligations.

The major area in which parents and therapists interact is the development of the Individualized Educational Program (IEP) for the child. In poorly run programs, the process is usually painful for the parents because they are subjected to the reports of the professionals in an arena-style conference. Parents usually leave the conference intimidated and more confused than when they went in. They, certainly do not come out feeling empowered. Andrews and Andrews (1993) presented a model for developing an educational plan that serves to empower parents, and I think this model needs to be widely adopted. In this approach, which is family centered, all members of the family are encouraged to participate. The professionals listen to the families and encourage them to participate actively in the child's assessment. Andrews and Andrews offered enabling techniques adapted from family therapy approaches that are readily within the grasp of professionals who work with persons with communication disorders.

Multiculturalism

In a fascinating article, Van Kleeck (1994) described the many cultural traps into which the insensitive speech–language pathologist can fall. For example, when the speech–language pathologist assumes that getting the child to initiate more communication means getting the child to initiate conversation with adults, he or she unwittingly may be violating a family norm. In many cultures, children are not encouraged to initiate conversations with adults. We must avoid imposing our cultural values on others. It is so easy to operate from our own ethnocentric perspective that we fail to appreciate cultural differences.

On the other hand, there is an equal danger that, in looking for cultural differences among populations, we fall into the trap of cultural stereotyping. Within any cultural grouping, there are always variations in behavior, and the generalizations we make about a population may not apply to the specific individual with whom we are working. We need to understand that in one sense we are all multicultural; each family must be approached as a marvelous experiment of one. We must take each family individually and allow its members to teach us the best way for them to learn. We always need to respect the dignity of each family we encounter, and as Van Kleeck (1994) pointed out, we must create an educational program to fit the family rather than try to fit the family to our program. This notion supports everything that is in this text. By listening to and valuing our clients, we will always respect their unique cultural heritage.

The Limits of Counseling

In a thoughtful article, Stone and Olswang (1989) tried to define the boundaries for counseling by speech–language pathologists and audiologists. They argued that many times the problem is not that we need better counseling skills but that the client should be referred to a mental health professional. The boundary for this referral is very hard to define, and Stone and Olswang failed to offer clear guidelines. I am not sure I can offer any either. I have found that as I become more comfortable with myself and more comfortable with affect in my relationships, my professional boundaries have expanded and I am willing to allow my professional relationships much greater latitude. I find myself less willing to refer clients. It is very difficult to refer a client to a mental health professional in such a way that does not provoke extreme anxiety in the client. The message you are sending to the client, no matter how nicely put, is that the problem is so formidable that he or she needs to see someone else. This often is very threatening to clients.

In actuality, in that situation the person with the problem often is the speech–language pathologist or audiologist. I think psychologists and social workers who are employed in clinics need to provide ongoing inservice training to speech–language pathologists/audiologists to help them improve their counseling skills and confidence in their ability to relate on the affect level with clients. This requires the mental health professional to be professionally secure and able to accept a consultative role. Unfortunately, there are many Annie Sullivan psychologists and social workers who are anxious to rescue the speech–language pathologist/audiologist; this de-skills them in the same way that Annie de-skilled Mrs. Keller.

Undoubtedly, there are people with emotional disturbances who develop communication disorders or who are the relatives of someone with a communication disorder. These people are not just upset, although they may seem so at the beginning; they truly have emotional disturbances and a multitude of life-adjustment problems. I have a responsibility to identify these clients and then to set my limits. I do not refer clients to mental health professionals because I don't presume to know what is best for someone else. However, I have clear boundaries for myself, and I will tell clients that I do not feel professionally comfortable counseling them and do not want to delve further. Clients then generally refer themselves for further counseling. If they ask me for a referral, I am able to give them the names of two or three people with whom to consult; I won't make the choice for them.

Counseling skills permeate everything I do. I do not want or expect to charge for "counseling." This is something a mental health professional does, and it would be an inappropriate professional invasion if I did it. Speech–language pathologists and audiologists need to infuse counseling concepts in everything they do. Many of the problems we encounter with clients can be solved by using techniques culled from the family therapy literature. For example, Stone (1992) demonstrated how a systems approach could be used to analyze problematic relationships to improve the interactions between the professional and the families involved in the therapy. As mentioned previously, Andrews and Andrews (1993) used system theory to help empower families during the IEP process. I think this trend will continue as we discover and use material and techniques garnered from the psychotherapy literature.

I think the key to counseling is the congruence of the counselor. As I become more congruent, technique slips away or, more accurately, becomes incorporated into everything I do. The most important thing a counselor brings to the helping relationship is self. The importance of the congruent professional far exceeds the value of any diagnostic test or specific techniques in counseling. If the literature on the desirable personality characteristics of the counselor were examined, it would appear that no one would qualify unless one could also qualify for sainthood. It is not necessary to be an entirely self-actualized person to be an effective counselor; rather, I think one needs to have a deep interest in people and a sensitivity to others. One needs to be a caring individual who does not impose beliefs on others, who maintains a constant awareness of self, and who does not hide behind the artificiality of being a professional. Professional growth will be measured by how we grow as individuals. We owe our profession and our clients the commitment to learn about ourselves as well as our field; we can do no less.

REFERENCES

Albertini, J., Smith, J., & Metz, D. (1983). Small group versus individual speech therapy with hearing impaired young adults. *Volta Review, 85*, 83–87.

Alpiner, J. (1978). Ancillary personnel in rehabilitation. In S. Alpiner (Ed.), *Handbook of adult rehabilitative audiology* (pp. 232–274). Baltimore: Williams & Wilkins.

Andrews, M. A. (1986). Application of family therapy techniques to the treatment of language disorders. *Seminars in Speech and Language, 7*, 347–358.

Andrews, M., & Andrews, J. (1993). Family-centered techniques: Integrating enablement into the IFSP process. *Journal of Childhood Communication Disorders, 15*(1), 41–46.

Arbuckle, D. S. (1970). *Counseling: Philosophy, theory and practice* (2nd ed.). Boston: Allyn & Bacon.

Asha Interview: Geri Jewell. (1983). *Asha, 25*, 18–22.

Atkins, D. (Ed.). (1987). Families and their hearing impaired children. *Volta Review, 89* (Monograph No. 5).

Backus, O., & Beasley, J. (1951). *Speech therapy with children*. Cambridge, MA: Houghton Mifflin.

Bardach, J. (1969). Group sessions with wives of aphasic patients. *International Journal of Group Psychotherapy, 119*, 361–366.

Baumgarten, M., Battista, R., Infante-Rivard, M., Hanley, J., Becker, R., & Gauthier, S. (1990). The psychological and physical health of family members caring for an elderly person with dementia. *Journal of Clinical Epidemiology, 45*(1), 61–70.

Beavers, R., & Voeller, M. (1983). Comparing and contrasting the Olson Circumplex Model with the Beavers Systems Model. *Family Process, 22*, 85–98.

Berry, J. O. (1987). Strategies for involving parents for young children using augmentative and alternative communication. *Augmentative and Alternative Communication, 3*(2), 90–93.

Bodner, B., & Johns, J. (1977). Personality and hearing impairment: A study in locus of control. *Volta Review, 79*, 362–368.

Boorstein, S. (1996) *Transpersonal psychotherapy*. Albany: State University of New York Press.

Bynner, W. (Trans.). (1962). *The way of life according to Lao-tzu*. New York: Capricorn Books.

Caracciolo, G., Rigrodsky, S., & Morrison, E. (1978). A Rogerian orientation to the speech–language pathology supervisory relationship. *Asha, 20*, 286–290.

Cartwright, L., & Ruscello, D. (1979). A survey on parent involvement in speech clinics. *Asha, 21*, 275–280.

Cassell, E. (1991). *The nature of suffering*. New York: Oxford University Press.

Cohen, M. (1996) *Dirty details*. Philadelphia: Temple University Press.

Cole, S., O'Conner, S., & Bennett, L. (1979). Self-help groups for clinic patients with chronic illness. *Primary Care, 6*(2), 325–339.

Coles, R. (1970). *Erik H. Erikson: The growth of his work*. Boston: Little, Brown.

Cook, J. (1964). Silences in psychotherapy. *Journal of Counseling Psychology, 11*, 42–46.

Cooper, E. (1966). Client–clinician relationships and concomitant factors in stuttering therapy. *Journal of Speech and Hearing Disorders, 9,* 194–199.

Cottrel, A., Montague, J., Farb, J., & Throne, S. (1980). An operant procedure for improving vocabulary definition performance in developmentally delayed children. *Journal of Speech and Hearing Disorders, 45,* 90–95.

Craig, A., Franklin, J., & Andrews, G. (1985). The prediction and prevention of relapse in stuttering. *Behavior Modification, 9,* 422–442.

Crandall, C. (1997) An update on counseling instruction within audiology programs. *Journal of the Acadamy of Rehabilitative Audiology, 30,* 1–10.

Crane, S., & Cooper, E. (1983). Speech–language clinician personality variables and clinical effectiveness. *Journal of Speech and Hearing Disorders, 48,* 140–147.

Crowley, M., Keane, K., & Needham, C. (1982). Fathers: The forgotten parents. *American Annals of the Deaf, 127,* 38–45.

Culatta, R., Colucci, S., & Wiggins, E. (1975). Clinical supervisors and trainees: Two views of a process. *Asha, 171,* 152–156.

Culpepper, B., Mendel, L., & McCarthy, P. (1994). Counseling experience and training offered by ESB-accredited programs. *Asha, 36,* 55–64.

Dale, P. (1991). The validity of a parent report measure of vocabulary and syntax at 24 months. *Journal of Speech and Hearing Research, 34,* 565–571.

Darius, B. (1988). *A study of siblings of hearing impaired children: How they were affected by the handicap.* Unpublished master's thesis, Emerson College, Boston.

Davies, H., Priddy, M., & Tinkleberg, J. (1986). Support groups for male caregivers of Alzheimer's patients. *Clinical Gerontologist, 5,* 385–394.

Dee, A. (1981). Meeting the needs of the parents of deaf infants. *Language, Speech and Hearing Services in Schools, 12,* 13–21.

Dowaliby, E., Burke, N., & McKee, B. (1983). A comparison of hearing impaired and normally hearing students on locus of control, people orientation and study habits and attitudes. *American Annals of the Deaf, 128,* 53–59.

Dundon, M., Carmer, S., & Novak, C. (1987, March). *Distress and coping among caregivers of victims of Alzheimer's disease.* Paper presented at the annual meeting of the American Psychological Association, New York.

Edgerly, R. (1975). *The effectiveness of parent counseling in the treatment of children with learning disabilities.* Unpublished doctoral dissertation, Boston University.

Egolf, D., Shames, G., Johnson, P., & Kasprisin-Burrell, S. (1972). The use of parent interaction patterns in therapy for young stutterers. *Journal of Speech and Hearing Disorders, 37,* 222–227.

Ellis, A. (1977). The basic clinical theory of rational-emotive therapy. In A. Ellis & R. Grieger (Eds.), *Handbook of rational-emotive therapy* (pp. 11–19). New York: Springer.

Emerick, L. (1988). Counseling adults who stutter: A cognitive approach. *Seminars in Speech and Language, 9,* 257–267.

Emerson, R. (1980). *Changes in depression and self-esteem of spouses of stroke patients with aphasia as a result of group counseling.* Unpublished doctoral dissertation, Oregon University, Eugene.

English, K., Mendel, L., Rojeski, T., & Hornak, J. (1999) Counseling in Audiology; or learning to listen: Pre and post measures from an audiology counseling course. *American Journal of Audiology, 8,* 34–39.

Epstein, N., Bishop, D., & Baldwin, L. (1982). McMaster model of family functioning: A view of the normal family. In E. Walsh (Ed.), *Normal family process* (pp. 148–172). New York: Guilford Press.

Erikson, E. H. (1950). *Childhood and society* (2nd ed.). New York: Norton.

Farran, C., Keane-Hagerty, E., Salloway, S., Kupferer, S., & Wilken, C. (1991). Finding meaning: An alternative paradigm for Alzheimer's disease family caregivers. *The Gerontologist, 31*(4), 483–489.

Featherstone, H. (1980). *A difference in the family.* New York: Basic Books.

Fialka, J. (1994). *Advice to professionals who must conference cases* [poem]. Unpublished work.

Flahive, M., & White, S. (1982). Audiologists and counseling. *Journal of the Academy of Rehabilitative Audiology, 10,* 275–287.

Fleming, M. (1972). A total approach to communication therapy. *Journal of the Academy of Rehabilitative Audiology, 5,* 28–35.

Fromm, E. (1941). *Escape from freedom.* New York: Holt, Rinehart & Winston.

Gallagher, J. J., Cross, A., & Scharfman, W. (1981). Parental adaptation to a young handicapped child: The father's role. *Journal of the Division for Early Childhood, 3,* 3–14.

Gardner, H. (1991). *The unschooled mind.* New York: Basic Books.

Gath, A. (1977). The impact of the abnormal child upon the parents. *British Society of Psychiatry, 130,* 405–410.

Girolametta, M. E., Greenberg, J., & Manolson, A. (1986). Developing dialogue skills: The Hanen early language parent program. *Seminars in Speech and Language, 7,* 367–382.

Gregory, H. (1983). *The clinician's attitudes in counseling stutterers* (Publication No. 18). Memphis: Speech Foundation of America.

Grossman, E. K. (1972). *Brothers and sisters of retarded children.* Syracuse, NY: Syracuse University Press.

Haas, W. H., & Crowley, D. S. (1982). Professional information dissemination to parents of preschool hearing-impaired children. *Volta Review, 84,* 17–23.

Hahn, T. N. (1998). *The heart of the Buddha's teaching.* New York: Broadway Books

Hallahan, P., Gasar, A., Cohen, S., & Tarver, S. (1978). Selective attention and locus of control in learning disabled and normal children. *Journal of the Learning Disabled, 11,* 47–57.

Hansen, J., Stavis, R., & Warner, R. (1977). *Counseling theory and process.* Boston: Allyn & Bacon.

Harris, S., Handiman, J., & Palmer, C. (1985). Parents and grandparents view the autistic child. *Journal of Autism and Developmental Disorders, 15,* 125–135.

Harvey, M. (1989). *Psychotherapy with deaf and hard of hearing persons: A systemic model.* Hillsdale, NJ: Erlbaum.

Hinkle, S. (1991). Support group counseling for the caregivers of Alzheimer's disease patients. *The Journal for Specialists in Group Work, 16*(3), 185–190.

Hoffman, L. (1981). *Foundations of family therapy.* New York: Basic Books.

Holt, J. (1964). *How children fail.* New York: Dell.

Hornyak, A. (1980). The rescue game and the speech–language pathologist. *Asha, 22,* 86–94.

Israelite, N. K. (1986). Hearing impaired children and the psychological functioning of their normal hearing siblings. *Volta Review, 88,* 47–54.

Johnson, W., & Croft, R. (1975). Locus of control and participation in a personalized system of instruction course. *Journal of Educational Psychology, 67,* 416–421.

Kabat-Zinn, J. (1994). *Wherever you go, there you are: Mindfulness Meditation in everyday life.* New York: Hyperion.

Kazak, A., & Marvin, R. (1984). Differences, difficulties and adaptations: Stress and social networks in families with a handicapped child. *Family Relationships, 33,* 67–77.

Kingsley, E. P. (1987). *Welcome to Holland.* Unpublished work.

Klevans, D., Volz, H., & Friedman, R. (1981). A comparison of experimental and observational approaches for enhancing the interpersonal communication skills of speech-language pathology students. *Journal of Speech and Hearing Disorders, 46*, 208–212.

Kommers, M. S., & Sullivan, M. D. (1979). Wives' evaluation of problems related to laryngectomy. *Journal of Communicative Disorders, 12*, 411–418.

Kopp, S. (1972). *If you meet the Buddha on the road, kill him!* Palo Alto: Science and Behavioral Books.

Kopp, S. (1978). *An end to innocence.* New York: Bantam.

Kornhaber, C., & Woodward, L. (1985). *Grandparents/grandchildren—The vital connection.* New Brunswick, NJ: Transaction Books.

Kubler-Ross, E. (1969). *On death and dying.* New York: Macmillan.

Lachar, D. (n.d.). *Minnesota Multiphasic Personality Inventory.* Los Angeles: Western Psychological Services.

Land, S. L., & Vineberg, S. E. (1965). Locus of control in blind children. *Exceptional Child, 31*, 257–263.

Lash, J. V. (1980). *Helen and teacher.* New York: Delacorte.

Lavell, N., & Keogh, B. (1980). Expectation and attribution of parents of handicapped children. In S. S. Gallagher (Ed.), *Parents and families of handicapped children* (pp. 48–72). San Francisco: Jossey-Bass.

Lear, M. (1980). *Heartsounds.* New York: Simon & Schuster.

Lerner, W. (1988). *Parents' and audiologists' perspectives regarding counseling.* Unpublished master's thesis, Emerson College, Boston.

Levine, S. (1979). *A gradual awakening.* New York: Anchor.

Levine, S. (1982). *Who dies.* New York: Anchor.

Lieberman, M., Yalom, I., & Miles, M. (1973). *Encounter groups: First facts.* New York: Basic Books.

Lloyd, L., Spradlin, J., & Reid, M. (1968). An operant audiometric procedure for difficult-to-test patients. *Journal of Speech and Hearing Disorders, 33*, 236–242.

Lobato, D. (1983). Siblings of handicapped children: A review. *Journal of Autism and Developmental Disabilities, 13*, 347–364.

Lowe, T. (1989). *Grandparents view the hearing impaired child.* Unpublished master's thesis, Emerson College, Boston.

Lund, N. J. (1986). Family events and relationships: Implications for language assessment and intervention. *Seminars in Speech and Language, 7*, 415–436.

Luterman, D. (1969). Hypothetical families. *Volta Review, 71*, 347–351.

Luterman, D. (1979). *Counseling parents of hearing-impaired children.* Boston: Little, Brown.

Luterman, D. (1987). *Deafness in the family.* Boston: Little, Brown.

Luterman, D. (1995). *In the shadows: Living and coping with a loved one's chronic illness.* Bedford, MA: Jade Press.

Luterman, D., & Kurtzer-White, E. (1999). Identifying hearing loss: Parents needs. *Journal of Audiology, 8*, 8–13.

Madison, L., Budd, K., & Itzkowitz, J. (1986). Changes in stuttering in relation to children's locus of control. *Journal of Genetic Psychology, 147*, 233–240.

Malone, R. L. (1969). Expressed attitudes of families of aphasics. *Journal of Speech and Hearing Disorders, 34*, 146–151.

Martin, E., George, K., O'Neal, J., & Daly, J. (1987). Audiologists' and parents' attitudes regarding counseling of families of hearing impaired children. *Asha, 29*, 27–33.

Martin, E., Krueger, S., & Bernstein, M. (1990). Diagnostic information transfer to hearing-impaired adults. *Texas Journal of Audiology and Speech Pathology, 16*(2), 29–32.

Maslow, A. H. (1962). *Towards a psychology of being.* Trenton, NJ: Van Nordstrand.

Massie, R., & Massie, S. (1973). *Journey.* New York: Knopf.

Matis, E. (1961). Psychotherapeutic tools for parents. *Journal of Speech and Hearing Disorders, 26,* 164–170.

Matson, D., & Brooks, L. (1977). Adjusting to multiple sclerosis: An explorative study. *Social Science and Medicine, 11,* 245–250.

Mattingly, M. A. (1977). Sources of stress and burnout in professional child care work. *Child Care Quarterly, 6,* 127–130.

Maxwell, D. (1982). Cognitive and behavioral self-control strategies: Applications for the clinical management of adult stutterers. *Journal of Fluency Disorders, 7,* 403–432.

McCarthy, P., Culpepper, N., & Lucks, L. (1986). Variability in counseling experiences and training among ESB accredited programs. *Asha, 28,* 49–53.

McKelvey, J., & Borgersen, M. (1990). Family development and the use of diabetes groups: Experience with a model approach. *Patient Education and Counseling, 16,* 61–67.

Meadow, K. (1981). Burnout in professionals working with deaf children. *American Annals of the Deaf, 126,* 13–19.

Mendelsohn, M., & Rozek, E. (1983). Denying disability: The case of deafness. *Family Systems Medicine, 1*(2), 37–47.

Miller, M., & Potter, R. (1982). Professional burnout among speech–language pathologists. *Asha, 24,* 177–180.

Minuchin, S. (1974). *Families and family therapy.* Cambridge, MA: Harvard University Press.

Minuchin, S., Rosman, B., & Baker, L. (1978). *Psychosomatic families.* Cambridge, MA: Harvard University Press.

Mitford, J. (1963). *The American way of death.* New York: Simon & Schuster.

Moore, P. (1982). Voice disorders. In G. Shames & E. Wiig (Eds.), *Human communication disorders* (pp. 312–346). Columbus, OH: Merrill.

Moustakes, C. (1961). *Loneliness.* Englewood Cliffs, NJ: Prentice Hall.

Munro, J., & Bach, T. (1975). Effect of time limited counseling on client change. *Journal of Counseling Psychology, 22,* 395–406.

Murphy, A. (1981). *Special children, special parents.* Englewood Cliffs, NJ: Prentice Hall.

Murphy, A. (1982). The clinical process and the speech language pathologist. In G. Shames & E. Wiig (Eds.), *Human communication disorders* (pp. 386–402). Columbus, OH: Merrill.

Nuland, S. D. (1994). *How we die.* New York: Knopf.

Olson, D., Russell, C., & Sprenkle, D. (1983). Circumflex model of marital and family systems: VI. Theoretical update. *Family Process, 22,* 69–83.

Pearlin, L., & Schooler, S. (1978). The structure of coping. *Journal of Health and Social Behavior, 19,* 2–21.

Peck, S. (1978). *The road less traveled.* New York: Simon & Schuster.

Pedersen, F. (1976). Does research on children reared in father absent families yield information on father influences? *Family Coordinator, 25*, 459–463.

Perkins, W. P. (1977). *Speech pathology: An applied behavioral science* (2nd ed.). St. Louis: Mosby.

Pickering, M. (1977). An examination of concepts operative in the supervisory process and relationship. *Asha, 19*, 697–770.

Post, J. (1983). I'd rather tell a story than be one. *Asha, 25*, 22–25.

Rabins, P. (1984). Management of dementia in the family context. *Psychosomatics, 25*, 369–375.

Rimm, D. C., & Cunningham, H. M. (1985). Behavior therapies. In S. J. Lynn & J. P. Garske (Eds.), *Contemporary psychotherapies* (pp. 44–70). Columbus, OH: Merrill.

Robertson, E., & Suinn, R. (1968). The determination of rate of progress of stroke patients through empathy measures of patient and family. *Journal of Psychosomatic Research, 12*, 189–193.

Robertson, M. (1999) Counseling clients with acquired hearing impairment. *International Journal for the Advancement of Counseling, 21*, 31–42.

Rogers, C. (1951). *Client centered therapy.* Boston: Houghton Mifflin.

Rogers, C. (1980). *A way of being.* Boston: Houghton Mifflin.

Rollins, W. (1988). Counseling spouses of the communicatively impaired. *Seminars in Speech and Language, 9*, 269–277.

Rosenberg, M. (1997) *The role of counseling psychology in the field of speech and hearing disorders.* Unpublished dissertation, University of Wisconsin, Madison.

Rotter, S. (1966). Generalized expectancies for internal versus external control of reinforcement. *Psychology Monographs: General and Applied, 1* (Whole No. 609).

Roy, R. (1990). Consequences of parental illness on children: A review. *Social Work and Social Sciences Review, 2*(2), 109–121.

Sabbeth, B., & Leventhal, J. (1988). Trial balloons: When families of ill children express needs in veiled ways. *Children's Health Care, 171*, 87–92.

Sager, C. (1978). *Marriage contract and couple therapy.* New York: Rawson, Wade.

Sandow, S., & Clarke, D. B. (1977). Home intervention with parents of severely subnormal, preschool children: An interim report. *Child Care, Health and Development, 4*, 29–39.

Satir, V. (1967). *Conjoint family therapy.* Palo Alto, CA: Science & Behavior Books.

Schein, J. (1982). Group techniques applied to deaf and hearing-impaired persons. In M. Seligman (Ed.), *Group psychotherapy and counseling with special populations* (pp. 41–60). Baltimore: University Park Press.

Schlessinger, H. (1994). The elusive X factor: Parental contributions to literacy. In M. Walworth, D. Moones, & T. O'Rourke (Eds.), *A free hand* (pp. 37–66). Silver Springs, MD: TS Publishers.

Schlessinger, H., & Meadow, K. (1971). *Deafness and mental health: A developmental approach* (Report No. RD283-S). Washington, DC: U.S. Department of Health, Education, and Welfare.

Schwirian, P. (1976). Effects of the presence of a hearing impaired preschool child in the family on behavior patterns of older "normal" siblings. *American Annals of the Deaf, 121*, 373–380.

Seligman, M. (1982). *Group psychotherapy and counseling with special populations.* Baltimore: University Park Press.

Seligman, M., & Lobato, D. (1983). Siblings of handicapped persons. In M. Seligman (Ed.), *The family with a handicapped child: Understanding and treatment* (pp. 3–27). New York: Grune & Stratton.

Shames, G., & Florance, C. (1982). Disorders of fluency. In G. Shames & E. Wag (Eds.), *Human communication disorders* (pp. 86–110). Columbus, OH: Merrill.

Shapiro, E. (1994). *Grief as a family process.* New York: Guilford Press.

Shirlberg, L., Diabless, D., Carlson, K., Filley, F., Kwiatkowski, J., & Smith, M. (1977). Personality characteristics, academic performance and clinical competence in communication disorders majors. *Asha, 19,* 311–315.

Shlien, J., Mosak, H., & Dreikors, R. (1962). Effects of time limits: A comparison of the psychotherapies. *Journal of Counseling Psychology, 9,* 31–36.

Singler, J. (1982). The stroke group: Planning for success. In M. Seligman (Ed.), *Group psychotherapy and counseling with special populations* (pp. 170–196). Baltimore: University Park Press.

Ski Hi, Communicative Disorders Institute. (1985). *Manual for home visits.* Ogden: Utah State University.

Skinner, B. E. (1953). *Science and human behavior.* New York: Macmillan.

Starkweather, C. (1974). Behavior modification in training speech clinicians: Procedures and implications. *Asha, 16,* 607–612.

Stech, E., Curtiss, J., Troesch, P., & Binnie, C. (1973). Clients' reinforcement of speech clinicians: A factor analytic study. *Asha, 15,* 287–291.

Stone, J. (1992). Resolving relationship problems in communication disorders treatment: A systems approach. *Language, Speech and Hearing Services in Schools, 23,* 300–307.

Stone, J. R., & Olswang, L. B. (1989). The hidden challenge in counseling. *Asha, 31,* 27–30.

Superior, K., & Leichook, A. (1986). Family participation in school based programs. *Seminars in Speech and Language, 7,* 395–414.

Tanner, D. C. (1980). Loss and grief implications for the speech–language pathologist and audiologist. *Asha, 22,* 916–922.

Vance, B. (1998) Stroke! This isn't the script I was writing! In W. Sife (Ed.), *Enhancing the quality of life* (pp. 149–160). New York: Haworth Press.

Van Kleeck, A. (1994). Potential cultural bias in training parents as conversational partners with their children who have delays in language development. *Asha, 35,* 67–76.

Van Riper, C. (1965). Supervision of clinical practice. *Asha, 7,* 75–78.

Venters, M. (1981). Familial coping with chronic and severe childhood illness: The case of cystic fibrosis. *Social Science and Medicine, 15A,* 289–297.

Ventimiglia, R. (1986). Helping couples with neurological disabilities: A job description for clinical sociologists. *Clinical Sociology Review, 4,* 123–139.

Ward, B., & Webster, E. (1965). The training of clinical personnel: A concept of clinical preparation. *Asha, 7,* 103–108.

Webster, E. (1966). Parent counseling by speech pathologists and audiologists. *Journal of Speech and Hearing Disorders, 31,* 331–345.

Webster, E. (1968). Procedures for group counseling in speech pathology and audiology. *Journal of Speech and Hearing Disorders, 33,* 27–35.

Webster, E. (1977). *Counseling with parents of handicapped children.* New York: Grune & Stratton.

Webster, M. (1982). *Hear, Here, Newsletter of the Canadian Speech and Hearing, 6,* 235–237.

White, K. (1982). Defining and prioritizing the personal and social competence needed by hearing impaired students. *Volta Review, 84,* 266–273.

Williams, D. M. L., & Derbyshire, J. O. (1982). Diagnosis of deafness: A study of family responses and needs. *Volta Review, 84,* 24–30.

Wright, D. (1969). *Deafness.* New York: Stein & Day.

Yalom, I. (1975). *The theory and practice of group psychotherapy*. New York: Basic Books.

Yalom, I. (1980). *Existential psychotherapy*. New York: Basic Books.

Yalom, I. (1989). *Love's Executioner*. New York: Basic Books.

Yarnell, G. (1983). Comparisons of operant and conventional audiometric procedures with multi-handicapped (deaf–blind) children. *Volta Review, 85,* 69–74.

Index

About the Author

David M. Luterman, EdD, is professor emeritus at Emerson College in Boston and director of the Thayer Lindsley Family Centered Nursery for Hearing Impaired Children. He has dedicated his career to developing a greater understanding of the psychological effects and emotions associated with hearing impairment. He has successfully translated this understanding into an effective model of counseling that allows for content and affect change, giving new meaning to the word "counseling." Dr. Luterman has lectured on counseling at conferences throughout the United States, Canada, and abroad. He is a fellow of the American Speech-Language-Hearing Association. Dr. Luterman is the author of *Counseling Parents of Hearing Impaired Children* (1979, Little, Brown), *Counseling the Communicatively Disordered and Their Families* (1984, Little, Brown), *Deafness in Perspective* (1986, College Hill Press), *Deafness in the Family* (1987, College Hill Press), *When Your Child is Deaf* (1991, York Press), *In the Shadows: Living and Coping with a Loved One's Chronic Illness* (1995, Jade Press), and *The Young Deaf Child* (1999, York Press).